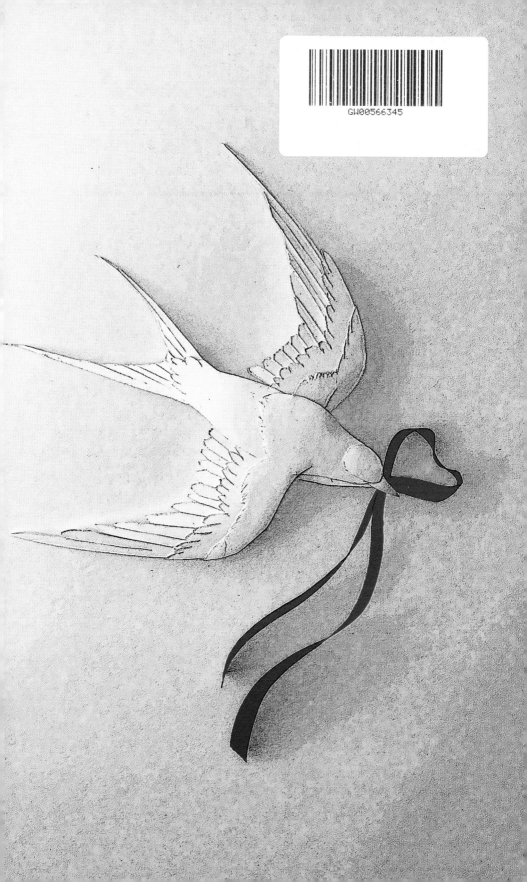

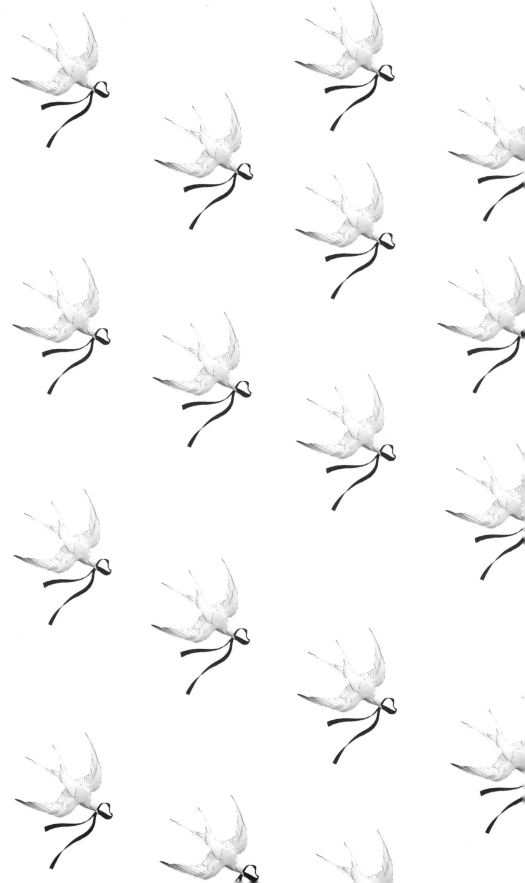

Love, Loss & Life

Real stories from the AIDS Pandemic
by Rupert Everett, Lord Fowler,
Jane Anderson & many more …

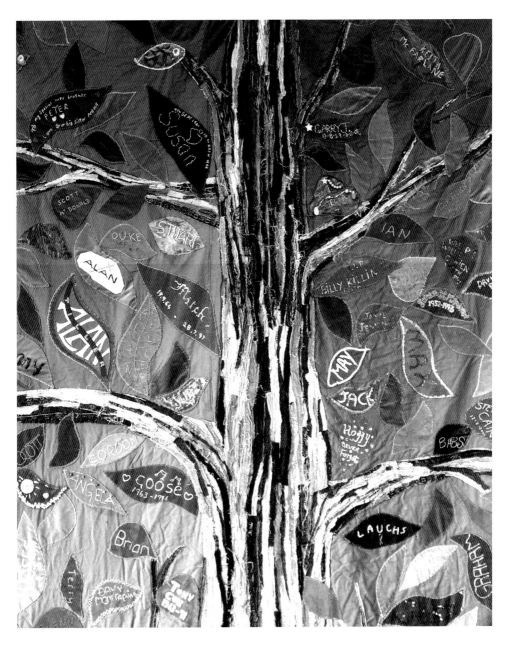

A detail from one of the many quilts stitched by friends and lovers in memory of those who died from AIDS and now collected by the AIDS Memorial Quilt Preservation Partnership.

Love, Loss & Life

Real Stories from the AIDS Pandemic

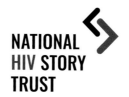

NATIONAL
HIV STORY
TRUST

First published 2021

Copyright © NHST 2021
The moral rights of the authors have been asserted.
These stories have been compiled by Nick Thorogood and Paul Coleman.

Access to quilt collection by kind permission of
© UK AIDS Memorial Quilt Conservation Partnership;
Sahir House; George House Trust; Positive East; Positively UK;
The Food Chain; Terrence Higgins Trust.
Quilt photographs © NHST

ISBN 978-0-9566561-7-9

A catalogue record for this book is available from the British Library.

Produced by Premium Publishing for
National HIV Stories Trust,
www.nhst.org

This project has been made possible with the provision
of a financial grant from Gilead Sciences Ltd

With Thanks to:
Cresta Norris, Sarah Andrew, Durell Barnes, Peter Wozney, Hannah Jones,
Julia Ellis, Andrew Hochhauser and the team at the NHST

Book design and layout by Amanda Helm
amandahelm@uwclub.net

Cover paper sculpture by Cheong-ah Hwang:
www.papernoodle.com and www.etsy.com/shop/papernoodle

Printed by Short Run Press Ltd,
Exeter, Devon EX2 7LW
www.shortrunpress.co.uk

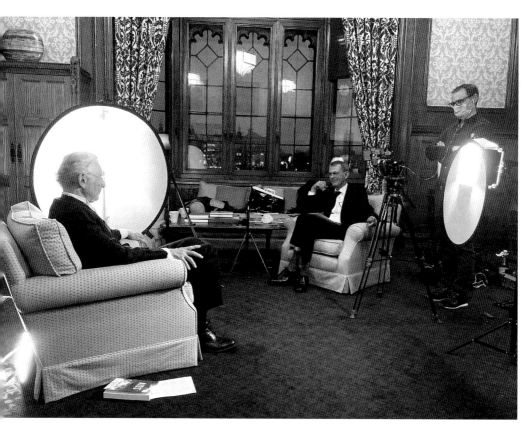

The National HIV Story Trust (formerly AIDS Since the 80s Project) filming an interview with Lord Fowler as part of the 150 hours of interviews reflecting on the AIDS pandemic of the 1980s and 1990s now housed at the London Metropolitan Archives. The archive will eventually be available for public access via the LMA.

As part of the archival process the interviews have been transcribed and form part of the contents of this book.

Having read the chapters in this book we hope you will visit the NHST website to find out more about our work and view samples of the interviews.

These interviews represent just a small collection from the archive, but reveal the silence and secrets of the time, showing how a community stood together and built a better future, even while it was being drained of life.

Contents

Timeline

Setting the scene:
Rupert Everett: "AIDS hit like a tsunami"

Part I: 1981–1992 "Half of you in this room will be dead…"

It was in the early 1980s that the world began to hear about an illness that seemed then to primarily affect gay men. In 1981 a serious case of pneumonia, Pneumocystis carinii pneumonia (PCP), appeared in five young previously healthy men in California. Simultaneously, in other parts of the United States, an aggressive form of cancer called Kaposi's sarcoma *affecting gay men was reported. By the end of the year, a rise and proliferation of deaths, in particular amont the gay population, was apparent and the scientific community was able to identify a correlation between the new condition with the immune system. Although they first referred to it as GRID – Gay Related Immune Deficiency – cases of PCP were also emerging among injecting drug users.*

By all accounts, HIV-1 probably originated in Central Africa, where the virus had crossed species from a chimpanzee. By the time those first cases were identified in California in 1981, there may already have been hundreds of thousands of people infected with the virus all over the world.

1981   **George Hodson: "Loss upon loss…"**
            David Eason: "A mad, terrible time…"
            Jonathan Blake: "To Life"

In December 1981, a gay man was referred to a London hospital with opportunistic infections indicative of a immunosuppression. In 1982, the Centers for Disease Control and Prevention (CDC) in the US used the term Acquired Immune Deficiency Syndrome – AIDS – to refer to the new illness. This was also the year in which the first cases of AIDS began appearing in Europe.

1982   **Winnie Sseruma: "Whole villages wiped out by Slim…"**

In 1982, at the same time, the medical community in Uganda reported several cases of people with AIDS. Researchers called the syndrome 'Slim', as weight loss and physical deterioration were the clinically dominant features of the condition. Central Africa has been the region with the highest prevalence of HIV. However, structural inequalities and deficient health interventions have contributed to largely disregard the response to the AIDS pandemic and its patients.

In 1983, several scientific advances helped to recognise what health services were up against. Researchers at the Pasteur Institute in France identified a new virus, the Lymphadenopathy-Associated Virus (or LAV), that could be the cause of AIDS. In November of the same year, the World Health Organization (WHO) who met to assess the global situation and began to monitor the number of cases throughout the world. By this time in the US, over 3,000 cases had been identified and, of those, 1,292 had already died. The following year the numbers had more than doubled.

1983/4   Professor Jane Anderson: "Dying before our eyes…"

In 1984 Dr Robert Gallo and his colleagues at the the National Cancer Institute discovered a retrovirus they called the HTLV-3, which was confirmed as the etiologic agent of AIDS. These advancements contributed to the development of a blood test to screen for the virus.

AIDS was then reported among the female partners of those diagnosed with the disease. It was realised that the virus was also being transmitted perinatally. The CDC ruled out transmission by casual contact, food, water, air or surfaces, and identified the major route of transmission as through blood, with the majority of cases being infected during sexual intercourse. They published their first set of recommended precautions for health workers.

In October 1984, bath houses and private sex clubs in San Francisco were closed due to high-risk sexual activity. New York and Los Angeles followed suit in 1985.

1985. From the earliest years of the AIDS pandemic, members of the gay and lesbian community, both in America and the UK, generated a diverse array of social movement organisations. These organisations developed their own support networks and mobilised political activism in response to the pandemic for receiving better care and treatment. In the UK, one of the earliest was the Terry Higgins Trust (later to become the Terrence Higgins Trust), a charity founded by friends of one of the first gay men to die of AIDS-related illness. It had been operating as a small voluntary organisation since 1982. However, in 1985 it was recognised that it was time to professionalise the charity and it set out to recruit its first two full-time paid employees.

1985   Nick Partridge MBE & Janet Green: "All in it together…"

1985 was also the year that the first high profile celebrity death from AIDS-related complications was announced, the actor Rock Hudson.

It had been known for some time in the US that haemophiliacs had also contracted the virus, but it was only in 1985 that blood banks began to screen the US blood supply. That year, a teenager in Indiana, Ryan White, who had haemophilia, was excluded from school because he had been infected with the virus through contaminated blood products.

Alan Burgess: "We didn't dare tell anyone."

By the end of 1985, every region in the world had reported at least one case of AIDS, with more than 20,000 recorded in total. The WHO had set up the first International AIDS Conference in Atlanta, Georgia. In 1986, the virus was renamed as human immunodeficiency virus (HIV). Although there were still no treatments available, the first antiretroviral medication, zidovudine (ZDV)– also known as azidothymidine (AZT)– would soon be approved. Nevertheless, much more was known then by health care professionals about how the virus was transmitted. Some schemes had already been set up to prevent people getting infected. For instance, Amsterdam in the Netherlands had pioneered the first needle and syringe programme to avoid sharing needles among injecting drug users. It was clear in the UK that a public health campaign could help lay to rest some of the myths about how the virus was transmitted, and save many lives.

Actor Ian Charleson, acclaimed for his role in the film Chariots of Fire, *dies in January 1990 aged 40. He was the first celebrity in the UK whose death was openly attributed to AIDS-related complications. He requested that the cause of his death should be made public. Fewer than two months earlier, with his face swollen by septicaemia, he had starred as* Hamlet *in Richard Eyre's production at the Olivier Theatre. It was considered one of the finest performances of the role ever.*

Ryan White, aged 18 – who had been banned from school in the US – died in 1990 from AIDS-related complications. In 1991, the year the red ribbon became a symbol to signify awareness and support for people living with HIV/ AIDS, Freddie Mercury announced that he was living with AIDS and died the following day. In the US, the basketball player Magic Johnson announced his retirement after being diagnosed with HIV. His subsequent campaigns on the subject helped dispel the widely held belief that the risk of HIV infection was limited to the gay community. Similarly, tennis star Arthur Ashe's announcement of his diagnosis through a blood transfusion in 1992 served to challenge stigma and demystify the condition. Although AZT had been approved for use as an antiretroviral drug in 1987, there was still no effective medical treatment for the virus. But change was on the horizon.

In June 1995, the FDA approved the first protease inhibitor which brought in a new era of combination antiretroviral treatment (cART). This novel medical treatment generated an immediate decline of between 60% and 80% in rates of AIDS-related deaths and hospitalisation in those countries which could afford it.

1995–98 Flick Thorley: "Some lived so long in the expectation they'd die, they couldn't cope with surviving…"

1997/98: In September 1997, the FDA approved Combivir, a fixed dose combination tablet of two antiretroviral drugs. This single daily tablet significantly improved the quality of life for people living with HIV.

1997–99 Adrienne Seed: "I felt entirely on my own…" Barbara von Barsewisch: "Some sort of healing…"

In 1999, the WHO announced that AIDS was the leading cause of death in Africa and the fourth worldwide. An estimated 33 million people were living with HIV and 14 million people had died from AIDS-related complications since the start of the epidemic.

Part III: 2000–the present

In July 2000, the Joint United Nations Programme on HIV/AIDS (UNAIDS) negotiated with five pharmaceutical companies to reduce antiretroviral drug prices in developing countries. In June 2001, the United Nations (UN) General Assembly called for the creation of a "global fund" to support efforts by countries and organisations towards ending AIDS through prevention, treatment and care. In November, the World Trade Organization (WTO) announced the Doha Declaration which allowed developing countries to manufacture generic medications in response to public health crises, like the AIDS pandemic.

2001   Krishen Samuel: HIV+ from South Africa

In January 2010, the travel ban preventing people living with HIV from entering the US was lifted. In July, the CAPRISA 004 microbicide trial was hailed a success after results showed that the microbicide gel reduces the risk of HIV infection in women by 40%. Results from the iPrEx trial showed a reduction in HIV acquisition of 44% among men who have sex with men who took pre-exposure prophylaxis (PrEP). In July 2012, the FDA approved PrEP for HIV-negative people to prevent the sexual transmission of HIV. PrEP was made routinely available via the NHS in October 2020.

For the first time ever, more than half of the global population living with HIV are receiving effective medical treatment, a record of 19.5 million people. Organisations around the world endorse the "Undetectable = Untransmittable"(U=U) message. This anti-stigma initiative launched by the Prevention Access Campaign signifies that people living with HIV who have adhered to treatment and achieved an undetectable viral load cannot sexually transmit the virus to others.

Afterword

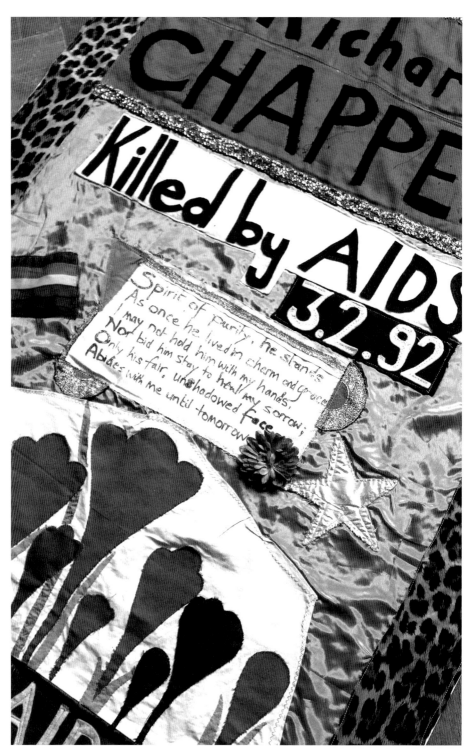

Detail from one of the fabric panels collected by the AIDS Memorial Quilt Preservation Partnership.

Foreword
Dame Erica Pienaar DBE, FRSA

Throughout my career in Education, I have been fascinated by the process of learning. I believe that the personal experiences of individuals and communities powerfully contribute to our learning and our understanding of the world we live in. Hence my enthusiasm to be involved with the National HIV Story Trust.

The word "history" and the English word "story" both originate from the Latin: "historia" meaning a narrative or account of past events. History could therefore be described as a collection of stories about the past. The transcripts shared in this book are a gift from the survivors of HIV.

Their stories reflect the experiences of men, women, trans, gay and straight, of all races.

These transcripts are an invaluable record of the experiences of those affected by HIV/AIDS and, most importantly, these personal narratives offer primary evidence of the AIDS epidemic of the 1980s and 1990s. They give us all an opportunity to reflect on the tragedy and compassion of the epidemic and to ask ourselves why it seems to have become almost invisible or even erased from history.

It is my hope that the gift of these transcripts will help us to understand the past, whilst living in the present and planning for the future.

Dame Erica Pienaar DBE, FRSA,
Freeman of Lewisham and of the
Worshipful Company of Leathersellers

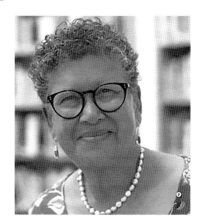

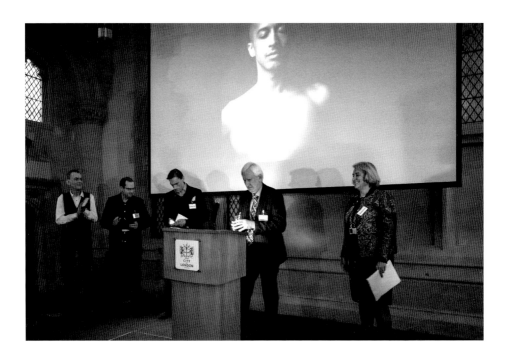

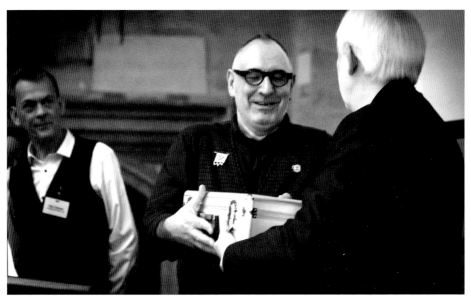

Jonathan Blake presenting the digital film footage of over 150 hours of interviews to the London Metropolitan Archives on 20th March 2019 at the City of London Guildhall. The archive will be open to the public for research access and as a record of social history in perpetuity.

Introduction
Paul Coleman
Co-founder of NHST

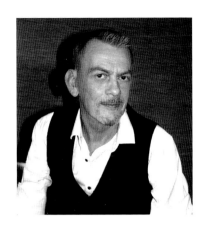

"To survive, you must tell stories."
– the words of the philosopher and novelist Umberto Eco.

Stories matter. History is more than a collection of dry facts and dates – the stuff of *real* history is people's lived experience, told and remembered to help shape our view of the past and to prepare for the future. Personal testimony becomes all the more important when it can cut through the fog of fake news, rumour, prejudice and falsehood.

This book is full of stories: the stories of those who died in the HIV/AIDS pandemic during the 1980s and 1990s; the stories of those who contracted the virus and lived; the stories of those who cared for them as doctors and nurses, or as volunteers and workers for the many charities that sprang up to help. These are stories of despair and hope that sometimes outrage, sometimes inspire and sometimes move the reader to tears. Above all, they are about survival in every sense of the word. You will find in the following pages stories of people who battled desperately to live, against the odds; stories of those who encountered destructive and negative reactions to their status; of those damaged by experimental drug regimes of the 1980s and 1990s; those who continue to suffer acute and complex PTSD; those who lost their loved ones, their jobs, their homes, their hopes. But these do not eclipse the stories of the milk of human kindness or activist-led initiatives that shaped a better world for those living with the virus.

We set up the National HIV Story Trust with one simple aim – to allow those who were touched by the AIDS pandemic in the 1980s, 1990s and 2000s to tell their personal stories of how those years affected them and their friends, and to preserve them for future generations. We started by filming and recording more than a hundred interviews with men and women who had been diagnosed HIV positive or been close to those who contracted the virus, as friends, carers, or medical professionals. Samples of those interviews are available to watch through our website and are also stored with the London Metropolitan Archives, so that future historians, researchers and the public will always have access to them.

But this year, 2021, marks 40 years since the first cases of what came to be known as AIDS were reported and recognised in America. It was the start of what the world came to recognise as a global pandemic, though it is now believed the virus had been circulating at a low level for many years before. To mark the anniversary, we felt we should find another way to use this important archive of personal testimony. Hence this book, which contains a representative selection of the many people we interviewed, telling their stories in written form.

It is perhaps ironic that we should find ourselves publishing the book in a year when the world is only just seeing the glimmerings of recovery from another global pandemic, albeit a very different one. But look closely at these stories and you may find some parallels: an initial and fatal lack of response from governments, along with a disregard for those most vulnerable to the disease; rumour and fake news circulating; prejudice against those seen as the source of the virus; the mobilisation of ordinary communities to support and help those at risk and extraordinary efforts by some in the scientific community to throw research protocols to the wind and rapidly find a way to treat or prevent the spread of the virus.

HIV/AIDS was, however, a very different kind of pandemic. As you will hear in many of the stories that follow, in Western countries it was initially perceived to affect just one group of people, gay men, who were as a result treated in many quarters with fear and loathing. This book focuses in some detail on their lived experience of the pandemic, which has been arguably the most significant event in modern day LGBTQ+ life, continuing to affect the community and its history today. AIDS probably advanced gay rights more than anything else in history and many of the freedoms the LGBTQ+ community enjoy today are due to changes instigated through the AIDS pandemic. Moreover, it changed the way that people were cared for and died and it changed the way all of us live now.

But although the LGBTQ+ community has been central in Britain to the story, this project is wholly diverse, reflecting the experiences of men, women, trans, gay and straight, of all races, UK born and migrant. It also reflects the experiences of those infected through blood transfusion. We should not forget that worldwide, more women and girls (53%) are living with HIV than men, nor that everyone has their own experience of the virus.

Nor should we forget that while the main focus of the stories in this book is the past, HIV is still very much with us. There have been some amazing advances in the treatment and prevention of the spread of the virus in the last couple of decades, but there are still many millions who are HIV positive, some of whom may not yet be aware that they are infected. HIV and AIDS remains a threat, particularly if we try to dismiss it as a pandemic that is 'over'. And for those living with the long-term effects of both the virus and its treatment, damage that can be psychological as well as physical, there are further issues. At the time of writing, the Infected Blood Inquiry in the UK continues and is far from its conclusion.

We have arranged this book to follow a loosely chronological structure and to offer an idea of the timeframe, we set the personal stories in the wider context of global developments in the progress and treatment of HIV/AIDS. The first part deals mainly with the 1980s and very early 1990s, as people in Britain began to grasp the enormity of this new virus. Both George Hodson and David Eason found themselves, in effect, at 'Ground Zero', living temporarily in the United States at the time of the first reports of an immune deficiency condition striking the gay community there … though as Winnie Sseruma reveals in her story, it was already circulating heterosexually in both men and women, under a different name, in Uganda and other African countries. We cover the first attempts by doctors in the UK to understand and treat the condition; Lord Fowler, Secretary of Health in the mid-1980s, describes the effort from the government to find a way to warn people about it; and how the infected blood scandal led to haemophiliacs and others treated with contaminated blood products to contract AIDS.

The second part of the book covers the scientific advances of the 1990s in understanding and treating HIV/AIDS, through the testimony of doctors and nurses whose careers became defined by their determination to help people with HIV. But the pandemic at this stage was far from under control, and the treatments were often brutal and physically damaging, as the accounts of those diagnosed and treated in the 1990s reveal.

The final section focuses mainly on the last 20 years or so, through the stories of people who have been infected more recently with HIV. It also revisits the stories of two of those infected in the first wave who appeared in Part I, George Hodson and David Eason, who are eloquently frank about the difficulties of ageing with HIV.

One of the authors in that part of the book, a young South African man diagnosed as HIV positive in 2009, writes: "Never forget those who died, because their stories are part of the history that binds us and takes us forward into the future." I couldn't agree more. This book represents many things: a memorial to lives that were lost, a celebration of what was achieved, a thank you to those who gave help and support to people with HIV and AIDS, a wake-up call for future generations and, above all, a testament to survival and hope for the future.

Read it, and remember.

Paul Coleman

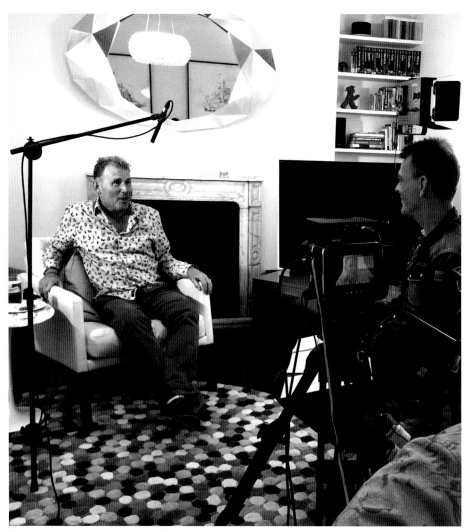

On location filming one of the 100 interviewees included in our archive and also housed at the London Metropolitan Archives.

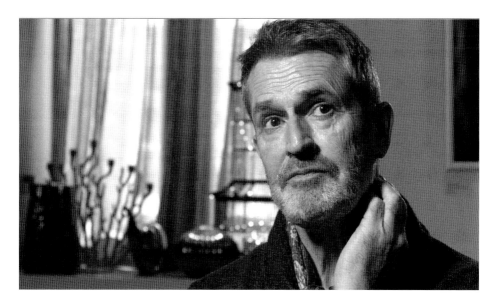

"This was when I first heard about the Gay Cancer. I turned on the telly one night and a boy's face appeared. He was someone I had been sleeping with on and off for years. In that split second before the sound came up, I knew. He was one of the early cases. Nothing would ever be the same."

Today we understand that HIV can affect anyone of any age, sex or race but back in the early 1980s it was a community of gay men who were first impacted by the virus to devastating effect. At a time when this community was just beginning to enjoy some freedoms, a sense of joy and some liberty, an even bigger challenge was on the horizon that would rip this sense of freedom apart and decimate a generation.

Here Rupert Everett reflects on gay life as it was leading up to the 1980s and how the landscape changed with the impact of HIV infection.

"Maybe we were in the middle of a revolution but we just didn't know it. For those of us that had survived the Seventies and were still here, something had definitely shifted."

Rupert Everett
"AIDS hit like a tsunami …"

On 5 February 2013, the British House of Commons approved the same-sex marriage bill in a landslide vote: 400 to 175. That night I was performing in *The Judas Kiss* by David Hare, a play about the life of Oscar Wilde.

It was an extraordinary evening to be playing Oscar – a man whose life was destroyed because he was a homosexual, with two years of hard labour for gross indecency, followed by three sad years of exile. Oscar died penniless in a cheap hotel in Paris. The dizzy heights from which he fell are hard to imagine for us today, but he was one of the great stars of the times. No party was complete without him, with three hits concurrently playing in the West End at the time of his arrest. Royalty attended his first nights, while later he supped with rent boys at Willis's.

Like many stars he felt himself above the law. As he waltzed into the fatal lawsuit against the father of his lover, he declared that "the working classes are behind me – to a boy". They weren't. Five short years later he was performing for drinks on the Parisian boulevard, with a missing tooth and a shabby suit. His companions were pickpockets and rent boys. He was a ruined man.

Doing the play that cold February night felt like surfing a historical wave. On the street, the *Evening Standard* was full of the news from parliament. The audience converged on the theatre with the same thought. Never was a play more suited to the times than *The Judas Kiss* that night. We were not just a hit show. We were a total eclipse.

The energy in the auditorium was intense. It felt – and I was not on drugs – as if the universe had briefly stopped in its tracks to watch. As I ran on for my first scene as Oscar, into the arms of Lord Alfred Douglas (played by Freddie Fox), I felt like the crest of a wave crashing on to the stage with all the blinding tragedy of gay history in my wake – the drownings, the burials alive, the hangings, the pillorying – all the tortures invented by man in the name of God. The applause was euphoric at the end of the show, as much for the day itself as for the performance. Finally, homosexual relationships were fully and equally accepted in law. We have come a long way. As Oscar predicted, the road to freedom has been long and smeared with the blood of martyrs, and the fight's not over yet.

I was sent away to school in the spring of 1967 at the age of eight. It is strange to think that on 27 July that year the Sexual Offences Bill received Royal Assent, and to be homosexual was no longer a crime. Technically. Based on the findings of the Wolfenden Report of 1957, the Sexual Offences Act decriminalised homosexual acts in private between two men over 21. (The law did not apply, by the way, to the merchant navy or the armed forces, to Scotland or to Northern Ireland. Those countries only decriminalised in the1980s.) To give one an idea of the national attitude, one has only to listen to Roy Jenkins, the Home Secretary at the time, during the all-night debate which led up to the vote. He declared that "those who suffer from this disability carry a great weight of shame all their lives". And he was on our side!

The Act did little to stop a steady rise in prosecutions, as the police took it upon themselves to raid clubs and bars, parks and bathhouses – anywhere public displays of homosexuality could be found or tricked out.

London in the mid-Seventies was still caked in soot, a postwar city of bedsits and mansion flats where the rich (hardly rich by today's standards) and the poor still rubbed shoulders. If you could sing for your supper, you could get by on £4 a week, crashing at other people's houses, eating at greasy spoons and vaulting the barriers at the Underground, with a spot of light grazing at Harrods if provisions were running low. Nobody worried about the future. Nothing was written down, so you found your way about using your nose.

Pretty quickly I sniffed out the forbidden city behind the crumbling façade of respectable Kensington. Following a man down the King's Road one night, I discovered a sex club called the Gigolo. With my heart in my mouth I descended a thin, rickety staircase – not knowing exactly where I was going, but following some interior sat nav, the same one that makes birds fly south, etc – into a writhing cavern of bodies under a naked red light bulb. "Rocket Man" was on the record player and I felt quite suddenly as if I had disappeared from my own life. There was a sense of complete freedom that I have rarely felt since. There was always the danger of the police and, of course, I had to be there on the night of the famous Gigolo raid. Suddenly the lights snapped on. Elton stopped singing as the needle scratched across the vinyl and the police swarmed down the stairs. There was mayhem as a hundred queens tried to pull their trousers up while being herded on to the street into paddy wagons.

Some attempted to run and were tackled to the ground and dragged back, but I just acted like a passing hooray and managed to squeeze through the crowd and get a lift to the Sombrero, where those of us who had evaded the police went to regroup and embroider the event into the annals of gay history. Being only 17 (the age of consent for homosexuals was still 21), I was living outside the law and I loved it. I felt I was a part of something, and I developed a passive distaste for the status quo, a sort of inverted snobbery, which I have never managed to shake off. The gay world of the late Seventies was a melting pot, classless and ageless. A decrepit duke in leather cruised a young plumber at the Coleherne while the smoothie from Sotheby's was the "sub" of a dangerous felon over the road at the Boltons. We were united just for being there, and sex was good for the fact of doing it. It didn't really matter who it was with.

I took my first trip to New York. I remember standing on the roof terrace of some rich queen's house in the West Village my first night there, dopey with jet lag, and looking across the rooftops at all those weird water towers perched on houses scribbled over with fire escapes against a backdrop of skyscrapers replete with Twin Towers blinking. The air tasted of metal. A couple of men were copulating on an old mattress on the roof opposite, observed by a half-naked lady riding the banister of her fire escape and stroking her breasts. Two men watched and tweaked each other's nipples in an open window. On another roof further off, a party of men danced on a tiny terrace, and disco music (helium screams over strings and a heartbeat) pulsed through the streets when I left the house. Men loitered on corners, still and tense as lizards, waiting to snatch at a tasty arse swishing by. I could hardly breathe with the excitement. The whole city seemed poised for the sexual act.

Emboldened by the success of the Stonewall riots of 1969, gay New York in the Seventies was a gritty and lawless jungle of sexual revelry. Queens like Andy Warhol, Halston and Steve Rubell ruled the Big Apple. Its constitution had been written at the Factory and on the dance floor at Studio 54, and it was all too good to be true.

But there was a strange feeling, as if one was being followed. Moving secretly through the misty dungeons and discos, the bathhouses and the rotting West Side piers, the invisible vampire was dancing with everyone, killing with a kiss: AIDS hit like a tsunami at the beginning of the 1980s. Many of the club cowboys lost their strut. They turned to skin and bone overnight, a new image of the bankrupt city, colour drained to black and white. They shuffled through the crowds wrapped in oversized scarves against the chill wind or a cold stare, but their glazed eyes and hollow cheeks gave them away. Parents held their children close as these queens limped by.

Meanwhile, back in the UK, I had become a West End star, playing a gay schoolboy groomed for treason in a play by Julian Mitchell called *Another*

Country. I mention this fact not to draw attention to my patchy career but because it was remarkable – a contradiction – that a story about boys falling in love with each other achieved commercial success during such conservative times. This was when I first heard about the Gay Cancer. I turned on the telly one night and a boy's face appeared. He was someone I had been sleeping with on and off for years. In that split second before the sound came up, I knew. He was one of the early cases. Nothing would ever be the same.

The next week we went to war.

A doctored poster of Ronald Reagan suddenly appeared all over America, plastered on walls at night by activists. He seemed to have Kaposi's sarcoma all over his face. It touched a nerve. Reagan had never once uttered the word "AIDS" in eight years in office. The organisation ACT UP took to the streets and – for the first time since Stonewall – when the police raised their batons the gays fought back. "Silence equals death" was their mantra. The television images were horrendous and surreal – young men streaming with blood being dragged from the steps of churches by policemen in spacesuits.

Women joined the fight, outraged by what they saw. Mothers stitched panels on to the AIDS quilt and took it to Washington, DC in a protest for their dead sons. The Princess of Wales walked into a hospital in Harlem and hugged a seven-year-old boy in blue pyjamas – AIDS and all – for the whole world to see.

The *Daily Mail* lit the fire that ended up as Section 28, reporting in 1983 that a book entitled *Jenny Lives With Eric and Martin*, about a little girl who lives with her father and his homosexual lover, was available at a school library run by the Inner London Education Authority. Conservatives roared with indignation at the idea of the "promotion" of homosexuality, especially since they bluntly considered us a disease trap. But despite the horror of AIDS, the tide was against them and it was not until May 1988 that Section 28 half-heartedly became law. Margaret Thatcher had misread the mood of the country. The night before the law was enacted, four lesbians invaded the BBC *Six O'Clock News* studio, one lady managing to chain herself to Sue

"But there was a strange feeling, as if one was being followed. Moving secretly through the misty dungeons and discos, the bathhouses and the rotting West Side piers, the invisible vampire was dancing with everyone, killing with a kiss ..."

Lawley's desk, only to be sat on by Lawley's male fellow newscaster.

Around that time two clever queens bought a sandwich shop in Old Compton Street, and suddenly Soho was claimed by the gay community. Gyms changed the gay silhouette and soon we looked much better naked than our heterosexual counterparts. A London club scene exploded at venues with strange names – FF, Queer Nation, Troll, Trade and the Daisy Chain. One popular song was called "Bring on the Guillotine", which always made me laugh. Maybe we were in the middle of a revolution but we just didn't know it. For those of us that had survived the Seventies and were still here, something had definitely shifted. Experience had toughened us. We began to have the same effortless confidence as straights. On the other hand, there was still no cure, but feelings of panic and helplessness were submerged in waves of hedonism that played out against a backdrop of hospital corridors and funeral homes.

In 1996 the first "cocktail" of antiretroviral drugs became available. Initially it was thought that this "combination therapy" could only buy time, but it quickly became apparent that the drugs were going to be a major game-changer. If you didn't become "resistant" and could tolerate them long enough (28 pills a day at various intervals – before food, after food, waking and sleeping) they could even turn around your "numbers" and – this was the elixir – render you "undetectable". For some it came just in time; for others, agonisingly close, but too late. Nevertheless, we were entering a new era tinged with optimism, where AIDS could be managed at least. As if in celebration, the following year Tony Blair won a landslide victory and I swept to Hollywood for my penultimate reinvention as America's singing and dancing gay best friend.

Today the world has gone full circle. Gay people seem to be doing all the decent things the straights used to do – getting married, having babies and recycling. I feel like an old grandmother, sitting in my rocking chair. The past is all twinkling lights on a snowy night.

So here we are, marriage material at last in one corner of the earth, while in the other we see the whole story repeat itself, in the destructive force of a world controlled by paranoid, petty dictators and so-called religious leaders – all men. It's public school all over again. Russia, Uganda, Greece and God are all putting their best foot forward to trample out the sin of homosexuality, so the revolution is not over. Maybe it never is.

―――――――

A version of this essay first appeared in the *New Statesman*. Rupert Everett is one of the 100 people whom the National HIV Story Trust interviewed on film to create the archive now housed at the London Metropolitan Archives.

Part I: 1981–1992
"Half of you in this room will be dead…"

It was in the early 1980s that the world began to hear about an illness that seemed then to primarily affect gay men. In 1981 a serious case of pneumonia, *Pneumocystis carinii pneumonia* (PCP), appeared in five young previously healthy men in California. Simultaneously, in other parts of the United States (US), an aggressive form of cancer called Kaposi's sarcoma affecting gay men was reported. By the end of the year, the rise and proliferation of deaths – in particular, among the gay population – was apparent and the scientific community was able to identify a correlation between the new condition with the immune system. Although they first referred to it as GRID (gay-related immune deficiency), cases of PCP were also emerging among injecting drug users.

By all accounts, HIV probably first emerged in humans as far back as the 1920s in Kinshasa in Africa, where the virus had crossed species from a chimpanzee. By the time those first cases were identified in California in 1981, there may already have been hundreds of thousands of people infected with the virus all over the world.

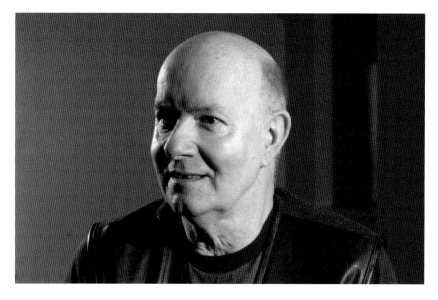

"I was drawn to San Francisco and … I found everything I'd hoped for …"

"It was two months of watching people die, wondering if I would be next. Every morning, a candle would be lit if someone had died in the night."

After a successful and lucrative career in advertising in his twenties, George Hodson spent two years in San Francisco studying photography and developing his own creative vision as an artist. Returning to advertising as a creative director, he lived in Hong Kong, Singapore and Thailand, before coming home to London where he was diagnosed with an AIDS-related cancer. Now in his seventies, he continues to work as an artist and breeds Griffon Bruxellois dogs.

George Hodson can legitimately claim to have been there at 'Ground Zero', living in San Francisco when the very first cases of HIV/AIDS began to appear among the gay community in America in the early 1980s. Diagnosed with AIDS himself a decade later, when there was still no effective treatment for the virus, he has somehow survived through several different cancers and a heart bypass operation into his seventies, but watched his lover, his friends and his fellow patients in the London Lighthouse dying of AIDS related illnesses.

George Hodson
"Loss upon loss …"

I have always been fiercely proud of who and what I am. I learned very early that I was homosexual and had my first love affair at boarding school when I was 16. But London in the 1970s was grey, dull and repressed and I was drawn to San Francisco and its exuberant experiment to build a community of gay people. So off I went down the Yellow Brick Road to see what was at the end of it, and I found everything I'd hoped for, a vibrant, joyous, celebrational, sexual Nirvana full of beautiful men holding hands. Businesses were run by gay people for gay people; the Sisters of Perpetual Indulgence, dressed as naughty nuns, were promoting gay politics. I became an honorary member of the Order, Sister Knickerbocker Glory.

In 1981, rumours began to circulate about a group of gay men in Los Angeles who, three or four months after a sex party, had all started to go down with what was being called 'gay cancer'. One day, I saw a Polaroid photo taped onto the glass at the front of the Castro Pharmacy, a close-up of a forearm with a purple lump and a rash. A sign underneath said anyone with symptoms like this should immediately go to the Gay and Lesbian Health Center. A shiver went through me; it felt like a portent of horrors to come.

I was invited by a friend to take photographs at a tea party he was holding – only when I arrived it became clear it wasn't going to be just a tea party. The whole room had black plastic on the floor. Within minutes of arriving, the guests began to shoot up with drugs and an orgy of heavy sex began. I fled in terror, because this didn't feel safe. It wasn't free love or intimacy, it felt like abuse; the experiment had gone too far and was out of control. Two weeks later, I left San Francisco for good.

Fast forward ten years or so, and I was living in Thailand with my partner, Sam. He was a gentle man like so many Thais, tall, handsome, with a black moustache, well-educated, a teacher of children with hearing difficulties at the American University in Bangkok. We were in many ways a perfect match. On a business trip to Hong Kong, I noticed a lump had formed on my belly. A

Chinese doctor said it was only a cyst but, by the time I returned to Thailand, it was growing and turning purple. I knew I had to go back to England for treatment – and within a week found myself in the Middlesex Hospital, on Broderip Ward, diagnosed with an AIDS-related non-Hodgkins lymphoma. The man in the bed next to me died in the night.

The day you get your diagnosis is like a personal earthquake. You had somehow to adjust your expectations, your opportunities, your desires, your needs, your sexual practices, your intellectual landscape. I'd lost, at a stroke, my lovely life in Thailand, my fabulously paid job, and had to leave behind my handsome lover and my gorgeous four-hundred-year-old house with servants and an orchid garden, all this replaced with a bed in a hospital ward filled with fear and grieving and screams in the night.

"The day you get your diagnosis is like a personal earthquake."

I then spent two months in the London Lighthouse residential unit, where I had chemotherapy. It was two months of watching people die, wondering if I would be next. Every morning, a candle would be lit if someone had died in the night. There were twelve of us in that unit and one morning there were three candles burning. I remember one beautiful young man who arrived on the ward and had tea with us in the living room. Then he stood up and told us he was now going into his room to starve himself to death. And he went into his room, closed the door and three weeks later, he died.

There's no single way to cope with a diagnosis of AIDS. Everyone has to do it their own way, and his way was as valid as the way I chose, which was to fight and go on fighting. Another man had a head swollen with purple lesions. He would get up every day, climb in his wheelchair and go downstairs into the restaurant. As he was wheeled in, every eye would be on him and the fear in the room was palpable, everyone knowing that the way this poor young man looked might soon be their fate too. But he held onto his dignity and was brave enough to eat in the restaurant every day. They were all heroes in their own way.

"They were all heroes in their own way."

There was a balcony where I went to sit every evening at six o'clock, alongside a very frail man with advanced AIDS. He was blind, he had dementia and was being eaten from the inside by Candida, a fungal infection. I never knew his name and we never spoke a word. But I'd take some strawberries with me, hold his hand, and very gently try to feed him a berry. He couldn't eat anything solid because the Candida had almost blocked his throat. And he would take the strawberry, and squeeze my hand. It wasn't long before he too was dead.

It was relentless, loss upon loss upon loss. Loss of people, loss of experience, loss of opportunity, loss of choice and loss of hope.

While at the Lighthouse, I was selected to have tea with Princess Diana on one of her visits. She was so beautiful that she shone, a good soul. She said: "Shall we play a board game?" I asked her which one she would like to play, and she said: "Anything but Happy Families."

As for my own family, I never really got on with my parents, but they came to visit me

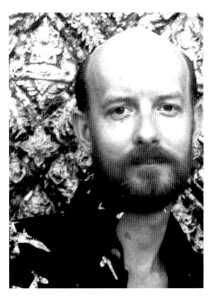

"There's no single way to cope with a diagnosis of AIDS. Everyone has to do it their own way …"

at the Lighthouse. The counsellors there told them they shouldn't be afraid of infection, so I was invited to have a meal at home with them. We had a stiff little dinner and I was itching to get away. As I was about to leave, I picked up my pudding spoon and noticed that on the back of it was a dot of red nail varnish. Looking closer, all my utensils had a red dot. I thought, that's it, we're done, and I never saw them again.

I fought to get Sam to be allowed into the UK to come and look after me. Chris Smith, the MP, took up our case, but it took a year, and when Sam arrived, he wasn't allowed to work and he wasn't allowed benefits. We were both living on about £60 a week. He was such a proud man, and I believe the fact he couldn't work depressed him so much it woke up the virus inside him – because, of course, he took a test when he came to Britain and he was positive. Against my advice, he signed up for AZT trials – I had refused to take part, because they were dishing out such huge toxic doses. Just as I was getting better from my cancer, he began to weaken and sicken and eighteen months later he was dead.

For the funeral, I cut some jasmine from my garden to wrap round his coffin, along with a beautiful hand-embroidered Thai silk scarf he'd once given me. I didn't want anyone else there in the church, just him and me, in silence, no words, just ten minutes together to let him go.

I still have his ashes which will be mixed one day with mine.

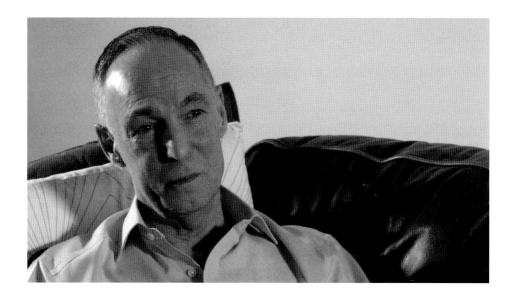

"Those were great years, with a terrific sense of freedom in the London gay scene, dancing into the small hours in nightclubs …"

David Eason volunteered at London Lighthouse helping to care for AIDS sufferers and, after this, with friends set up a number of initiatives to help people with the illness lead more normal lives, including the club-night 'Warriors'. He went on to become a complementary therapist.

"HIV seemed remote, nebulous, something we half-knew was happening over in New York and San Francisco, but still didn't fully understand how it would eventually touch us all."

David Eason was living in the United States when he first heard of a new illness affecting gay men. Throughout the AIDS pandemic he remained in touch with friends in the US, but also experienced the terrible impact of the illness in the UK when both he and his partner became infected. This moving account of the personal impact of AIDS ends with the death of his partner, but we will hear more from David later in the book.

David Eason
"A mad terrible time ..."

In 1982, I was a newly out gay man in my early thirties when the company I worked for sent me to Colorado in the US for a couple of months. It was there I first heard about this mysterious illness that was coming out of the West Coast.

I'll never forget the night it exploded dramatically upon my consciousness. A man with whom I was having a wonderful summer affair, Barry, worked for Public Health in Denver and he gave a talk at a gay man's social group, The Gay Business Association. He said: "There's something coming out of the West Coast, it's only affecting gay men, we don't know what it is, but there'll come a time when half of you in this room will be dead from it." As a social event, that pretty much killed the evening.

A couple of months later I was back in London and had put the mystery illness to the back of my mind, busy forging a new social life for myself in the UK. Those were great years, with a terrific sense of freedom in the London gay scene, dancing into the small hours in nightclubs like Heaven. I found a partner, Gary, who a few years later started work as cabin crew for Virgin Atlantic, his dream job. I was 33 and he was 24. We lived together right from the beginning in a stable partnership; it was my first real gay relationship. HIV seemed remote, nebulous, something we half-knew was happening over in New York and San Francisco, but still didn't fully understand how it would eventually touch us all. One day in the summer of 1983 I spotted a small advert in *Gay Times*, asking for volunteers for a cohort study into this new illness, to be carried out at St Mary's Hospital by the Wellcome Foundation. Some instinct flagged this up to me as important, so I joined the study and remained part of it throughout the 1980s. A couple of times a year I would undergo blood tests, psychological assessment and a whole battery of seemingly random tests – at this point I'm not sure anyone really knew what they were looking for, but it became an extremely valuable study as it threw up a great deal of useful data.

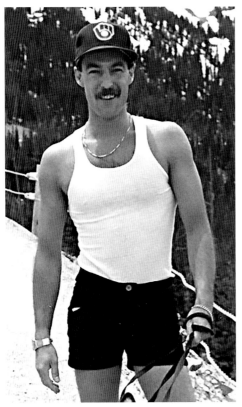

It wasn't until 1986 or 1987 that, for us in London, an undercurrent of fear started to creep in. I'd stayed in touch with my gay family in Colorado, especially Barry, and visited Denver often; the city was a gay hub, because of the mountains and the skiing. Barry's partner Horst was one of the first in Denver to become sick. Within a year or so I knew at least 20 people in the city who were positive. By then, it was becoming obvious that people in London too were affected.

One of the greatest tragedies of HIV is that, instead of treating it as a catastrophic medical pandemic, the rest of the world treated it as a moral issue. The attitude was that people who had it didn't matter, because they were gay and therefore expendable. They'd brought it upon

"One of the greatest tragedies of HIV is that instead of treating it as a catastrophic medical pandemic, the rest of the world treated it as a moral issue."

themselves: "It's your own fault if you catch it." But because the world didn't care about us, our response was: *We will just do what is needed and look after our own.* I went to volunteer at London Lighthouse, a place where so many went to die because they had nowhere else to go. Families would turn up from Scotland or the North of England, perhaps having just found out for the first time their son was gay, and now having to deal with the fact that he also had AIDS and maybe just a few days to live. They had no idea how to cope and the staff and volunteers helped as best we could. Once I remember sitting up for hours with someone whose lungs were affected, simply holding him upright so he could breathe more easily: as I say, we did what we could.

At that point, tests for the virus were not widely available, so generally people only discovered they were positive when they became ill. I was in the unusual position of knowing for certain I was negative, because I was part of the cohort study at St Mary's, tested twice a year. Then, one Bank Holiday weekend in 1990, I didn't feel well. My GP sent for an ambulance and I was taken into Hammersmith Hospital: I was seroconverting.[1] Six days later, my HIV test came back positive. As coincidence would have it, the consultant on duty there had been involved in the Wellcome study, knew me, and was dumbfounded. "I can't believe it," he said. "David, you were an all time negative in the study". When my partner, Gary, was tested two weeks later, he too was positive. He had never been tested previously and we had just assumed that he too was HIV negative. Apparently he wasn't.

It wasn't until 2020 that I discovered that, because I had remained HIV negative throughout the study period, out of the 400 gay men who were in the cohort, I was the only survivor.

Those were terrible times. Imagine reaching your forties, building your career with a close circle of friends you meet regularly for dinner parties – and then in the space of just three or four years, forty of them are wiped off the face of the earth. How are you going to behave? There's no manual for that. I had started a business from home, but was too distracted to keep it going. Work became secondary because, by that time, we were so busy caring for and burying our friends. I remember one particular chaotic week: friends of mine, Kevin and Chuck, had flown back from where they lived in Saudi Arabia because Kevin was ill. He was in hospital, and I sat with him as he lay dying. As soon as he had passed, I got on a flight to the States to see Barry and Horst. Horst was dying too but he'd been hanging on for me to arrive so Barry wouldn't have to deal with it on his own. He died a few days later and after his funeral I flew

"I had started a business from home, but was too distracted to keep it going. Work became secondary, because by that time we were so busy caring for and burying our friends."

1 When a person contracts HIV, the body starts to produce HIV antibodies. Seroconversion is the period of time when these antibodies become detectable and the person may experience flu-like symptons such as aching and fever.

"We knew he was going to die, and the only question was, do you do it badly, in distress and pain, or do you do it well, with your friends around you."

back to London and we buried Kevin. Chuck died the following year in his home state of California and Barry died in Denver in 1996. It was a mad, terrible time. Your perceptions change, and by the time I'd buried 25 or so friends, knowing that soon I would be burying more, I really couldn't summon the energy to answer the letters about bank loans and the mortgage repayments. We managed to sell the flat just before it was repossessed. Gary moved in with a friend and I went to the States to try and sort myself out. I'd only been there four months – this was December 1991 – when Gary phoned and told me he was getting sick.

Right from the day he tested positive in 1990, Gary considered it a death sentence, though at that point he was completely fit and healthy. Two years later he was dead. He was 33 years old.

During his last days, I lived at the hospital for three weeks, sleeping on a bed in his room. I ate the hospital food, but I bought his food from Marks and Spencer. It took every penny we had, but that's what you do. His lungs kept collapsing, and finally the thoracic surgeon, a tall, elegant, wonderful man, told us: "I'm really sorry, there's nothing we can do. The only option would be a lung transplant but you simply wouldn't survive the operation." Gary and I talked things over, knowing we didn't want to prolong this. We knew he was going to die and the only question was: do you do it badly, in distress and pain, or do you do it well, with your friends around you? We had a meeting to explain this to his doctors.

One asked Gary: "Anything we can get you?"

"A bucket of morphine," was his reply.

"A bucket of morphine coming up," said the doctor. We called Gary's family and close friends and told them they needed to be there in the next 24 hours. We dressed up the room, we put music on, and slowly increased the morphine to ease his pain. All through, we talked to Gary as if he were wide awake – just because someone is unconscious doesn't mean they

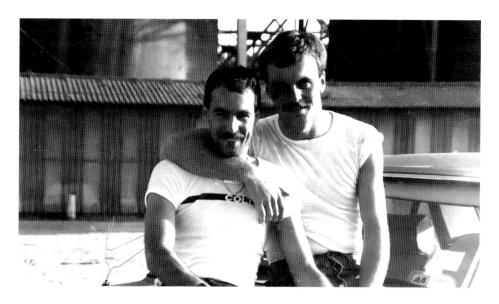

David and Gary, London 1983.

don't know what's happening. Once, when the music stopped, his close friend from Virgin Airways, Carol, who'd been given as much time off work as she needed to come and help us, asked what she should put on next. I said "ask Gary" – he hadn't spoken for several hours. She asked him – and he astonished us all by simply saying: "Enya." So we did.

Finally, peacefully, in the early hours of the morning, off he went. I'm proud of what we did for him. One of the nurses came in and helped me wash him and dress him, then I and a couple of close friends walked out of the hospital into a bright sunny morning, and I remember thinking: this is another dawn I'm seeing which someone I care about won't.

"I'm proud of what we did for him."

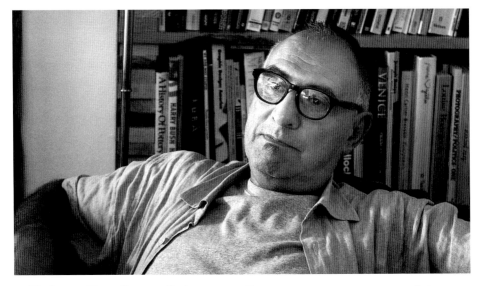

"To offer friendship and support is something very precious. When communities get to know one another, prejudice disappears."

Born in 1949, Jonathan Blake went to Rose Bruford Drama School, worked in theatre during the 1970s, and later became a costume designer with English National Opera, after being diagnosed HIV positive in 1982. The character of Jonathan in *Pride* was based on him, a film which told how a group of gay political activists, Lesbians and Gays Support the Miners (LGSM), formed links during the Miners' Strike in 1984 with a mining community in South Wales.

"Looking back to the 1980s, there was something really precious in the way the gay community came together in those years, to help others and to rally against a terrifying disease."

Actor Jonathan Blake describes the excitement of his youth when he first encountered the gay scene in London and San Francisco. His story is both delicious and dangerous and life was joyful. He tells how he had to rally against against 'a terrifying disease' and the world stopped. Jonathan reveals how the impact changed his behaviour, but his humour and exuberant love of life continues.

Jonathan Blake
"To Life"

When I watched *Pride* for the first time, it felt as if I had all the people from LGSM (Lesbian and Gay Men Support Miners) who are no longer here sitting on my shoulder and all I could do was think of them. It's not a film about AIDS, but it's impossible to separate that time in the early 1980s from what was happening in the gay community then. The film is full of images of people clasping hands and its message is that when communities come together, they can do anything – which is also for me the story of how the gay community itself responded to HIV and AIDS in those early years. We came together and we made a difference.

I knew very early on in life that I was different. As a small child, I had a crush on the school caretaker – I couldn't get enough of the scent of his body odour. Later, I went to a boy's boarding school and it was like heaven. Homosexuality was still illegal then, but the Sexual Offences Act in 1967 allowing homosexual acts between consenting adults came in just as I was heading to drama school. The age of consent for gay men was set at 21, but I didn't let that stop me. I spent every weekend around the Kings Road in London, in gay pubs – The Colville, opposite the Duke of York's barracks, The Coleherne in Earl's Court, a hangout for the leather brigade. There was Hyde Park, there was Hampstead Heath, there were parties and saunas and Turkish baths. I was a young actor and everybody wanted a slice of youth: it was all so exciting, but still very much on the edge, which was part of the frisson. The law only allowed homosexual acts between consenting adults in private. If you were at a club like Mandy's in Covent Garden, the bouncers would prise you apart if they considered you were dancing too close, because the club was afraid of losing its licence. If you took more than one person back to your flat, the police had the right to break down the door, and there were frequent raids on Hampstead Heath and other gay haunts. I decided to come out to my parents only once I was 21 – I feared they might shop me to the police for having underage sex – and on my birthday, at breakfast, I sat them down and told them. My mother said calmly: "But darling, we *knew*."

"Although the first cases of … AIDS had already been identified on the West Coast, no one really talked about it…"

"I was told I had a virus called HTLV-3, later renamed HIV, and that there was no treatment for it. It was effectively a terminal diagnosis."

My acting career was one of fits and starts, with long periods of 'resting' and waiting tables at Joe Allen's restaurant in Covent Garden which employed out-of-work actors. In the early 70s, I had some success in a BBC television series, *The Regiment*, so when some rich Americans I met invited me to New York, I could afford several months there, sampling the delights of the bath houses, at one point living in an apartment above the Continental Baths where Bette Midler started. The gay scene in the States was so much bigger and brasher and more hardcore than ours, and I was having a ball. But, in my heart of hearts, I knew I wanted to be an actor and to do that I would have to return to London.

By the early 1980s, I was still working at Joe Allen's in between acting jobs. Then a friend of mine was getting married in San Francisco, so I flew over for her wedding and spent a couple of weeks there, rooming with George Hodson. Although the first cases of what came to be known as AIDS had already been identified on the West Coast, no one really talked about it, and the life of the bathhouses seemed as extravagantly exciting as ever.

But back home in London in September that year, every lymph gland in my body erupted. I couldn't bear to hold my arms to my sides; my legs were agony. I had to give up my job at Joe Allen's and my GP referred me to the 'special' clinic at the Middlesex, suspecting syphilis. It wasn't. Shunted onto a side ward, where they put the gay men, in the bed next to me was an actor I'd met on tour and he was at death's door. I was told I had a virus called HTLV-3, later renamed HIV, and that there was no treatment for it. It was effectively a terminal diagnosis.

I turned in on myself. By December, I'd decided I might as well commit suicide. I'd cut myself off from my friends and was completely isolated. Everything I'd heard about AIDS convinced me I'd die a horrible death, so I planned to pre-empt it and slit my wrists in the bath, suitably medicated to avoid any pain. But I'm my mother's son, obsessively fastidious and tidy, and the thought of someone having to clean up after my messy death was so appalling that I couldn't go through with it.

I thought I would never reach forty, let alone pension age. So how did I survive when others didn't? So many died so quickly. Mark Ashton, the gay activist whose character also appears in *Pride*, lived for only ten days after he was told he had AIDS in 1987. Maybe it was sheer bloody-mindedness that preserved me. I reasoned that, since I couldn't kill myself, I'd better get out and live. I made myself go out again to gay bars and The London Apprentice pub. Then I saw in a gay newspaper that gay activists were organising an anti-nuclear pro-test around Greenham and Aldermaston. I'd always been politically committed, and though I feared I wouldn't know a soul, I hauled myself down to Gay's The Word Bookshop to catch the hired coach. The first person I saw was a guy in ochre and crimson pantaloons and wellington boots, with a shock of black hair. His name was Nigel Young, and he eventually became my partner.

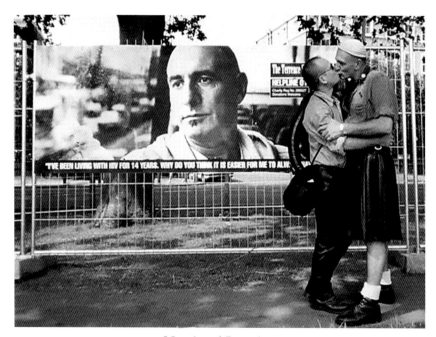

Nigel and Jonathan

By now I'd realised it was important to keep busy, because the more I kept busy, the less I thought about the virus. If you were out of work and claiming benefit, as I was, you could pay a pound and the GLC (*Greater London Council*) would fund you to do as many adult education classes as you wanted. I learned to make trousers and took a course on pattern-cutting – which eventually led to a job with the wardrobe department at English National Opera. And it was Nigel who persuaded me to join LGSM, which became in my case a kind of displacement activity to help me outrun AIDS. But at the same time, I felt passionately that the striking miners deserved our support. They were being harassed by the police, just as we gays had suffered constant police oppression.

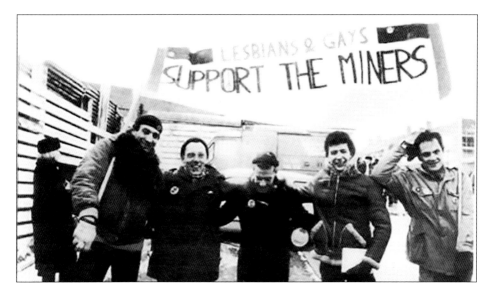

Wales 1984. Courtesy of © Lesbians and Gay Men Support the Miners (LGSM)

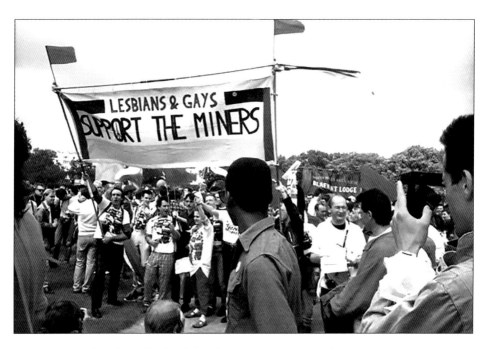

Jonathan at the Gay Pride March, Hyde Park 1985. Courtesy of © Colin Clews.

To offer friendship and support is something very precious. When communities get to know one another, prejudice disappears. It still blows me away that it was the South Wales miners who later pressured the National Union of Miners to use their block vote to put gay rights onto the Labour Party agenda, which brought about the lowering of the age of gay consent to 16 and civil partnerships. How extraordinary is that? Even more amazing to think *we* had a hand in it.

I refused to take part in the early drug trials for AZT in the 1980s – which the pharmaceutical companies were putting forward as a possible treatment – and I believe that too was a factor in keeping me alive. So many people were made worse by AZT, because doctors hadn't yet worked out how it could be used successfully, and I watched friends dying in agony. Fifteen years later, I finally gave in and underwent combination therapy, which made an extraordinary difference. Within a month, I went from being barely able to peel myself off the sofa to having the energy of giants, though like many others I paid a price: brutal side effects, such as peripheral neuropathy, where the nerve endings are shot.

Looking back to the 1980s, there was something really precious in the way the gay community came together in those years, to help others and to rally against a terrifying disease: the drop-in centres like the Lighthouse, Body Positive and the Landmark, where I volunteered; the extraordinary dialogue between patients and doctors that helped push forward treatment; the sharing of information that eventually gave us power over the virus. The genius of Steven Beresford, who wrote the screenplay for *Pride*, is that my character, a man with HIV, comes across in no way as a victim, and I'm proud of that. In too many dramas, the character with HIV is portrayed as the victim who is on their way to a sad end.

"But the more we can see people with HIV as normal, leading positive lives, the more we remove the stigma. For almost 40 years now, I've been HIV positive. I'm a good Jewish boy, and "L'Chaim" is a toast in Hebrew that means "to life." To survive is not enough. You have to get out there and live."

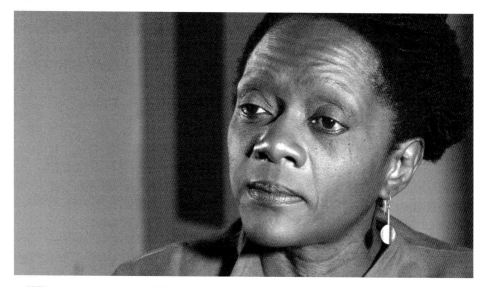

"Discovering I was HIV positive was a major shock that threw me utterly off-course. I was living each day as if it was my last …"

Winnie Sseruma was born in the UK of Ugandan parents, both teachers, who returned to Uganda and brought her up there. In 1981 she won a scholarship to go to the United States to study sociology at university in Kansas. After being diagnosed with HIV in 1988, she began to volunteer, supporting other people living with HIV, particularly among black African communities. She has gone on to expand her work internationally, working for Christian Aid and as a freelance consultant.

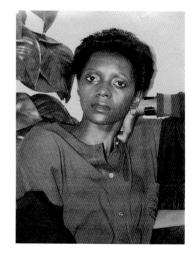

As a young woman, Winnie only gradually became aware of the word Slim, as AIDS was called in Africa, which was devastating communities in Uganda in the 1980s. When she was diagnosed HIV positive, she believed she was under a death sentence until she came to the UK and found both support and effective treatment. Her mission ever since has been to convince others that HIV need not be a barrier to living a full and fulfilling life.

Winnie Sseruma
"Whole villages wiped out by Slim…"

In Uganda, before I left for the US in 1981, there was talk of people growing very thin and dying through supposed witchcraft. But at that point I'd never heard of the condition, called Slim in Uganda, because people lost so much weight before they died. Uganda at that time was in turmoil: Idi Amin had been driven out of the country; Milton Obote was on the brink of power for the second time; the country was in chaos and almost on its knees. As is often the case in Africa, poverty, wars and lack of proper health care obscure what is really happening on the ground.

While I was in America, I started to hear through the media about a condition known as GRID: Gay Related Immunodeficiency Disease. At that stage in the US, there was little information on how it affected women, if at all. My university was run by Catholic nuns so we were, to some extent, in a protected little bubble. It was only when I returned to Uganda for a short time that I realised people were dying not only as a result of the war, but through this same condition. It was shrouded still in secrecy and mystery. At funerals, AIDS was rarely mentioned as the cause of death, which would be attributed to pneumonia or tuberculosis. Yet it was widely known that whole villages in East and Central Uganda had been wiped out by Slim.

During my visit home to Uganda, I dated a couple of ex-boyfriends without thinking much about it. At that stage, the mechanism of transmission for HIV was by no means clear. When I flew back to the States, I was to take part in an internship programme to get experience of social work. Anyone applying for such a position was required to be tested for various health conditions. When my results came back, I was told there were inconsistencies in my blood. They suggested further tests, one of which was for HIV. I had no suspicion I might be carrying the virus, so discovering I was HIV positive was a major shock that threw me utterly off-course. I was living each day as if it was my last, because I didn't know how long I could expect to live, and no one could tell me, since so little still was known about the illness. I was thousands of miles from

"I saw it as my role to support others living with HIV, especially those in the black African community, to persuade them they should seek testing and treatment."

my family, and didn't want to tell them because I knew it would worry them. Nor could I tell my friends, because you would hear conversations where people asserted that if they were sitting in a group with someone who had HIV, they would get up and leave.

I remained utterly isolated for six years, during which my younger brother in Uganda died of HIV-related TB. Soon after, both parents died of cancer, so half my family was gone. The counsellor I was seeing in the US, who disclosed he was HIV+, died too. I felt it would soon be my turn, so in 1994 I went home to Uganda to die, to save my siblings the cost of flying my body home.

As she was helping to unpack my luggage, my sister spotted my HIV medication – in those early days I was on AZT and DDI. She hid her shock and anxiety, and told me that she had friends living with the virus who knew private clinics that could help if I got sick. Before long, I almost had my wish of dying in Uganda, as I went down in quick succession with pneumonia, TB and really bad diarrhoea, but my great good fortune was that I could afford good care then and an HIV clinic kept me alive.

Two years later I left for the UK, to visit another brother. I had run out of HIV medication some time before because I could no longer afford it (it was not available in Uganda at the time) and this was meant to be just a short visit to recuperate. While there, I decided to get myself checked out at Newnham General Hospital. The doctor broke the news that I had a CD4 count of one[1], which meant I had AIDS. I was devastated – now I was certain I would die. But my brother knew someone with HIV who went to a local support group, Body and Soul. It was the first support group I had ever come across and I found 60 or so other women there living with the virus, all of whom were now on combination therapy and miraculously recovered as a result. It was an awakening of sorts. I decided there and then I should stay in the UK and, I hoped, to get better in a way that was not possible at that time in Africa.

I volunteered at Body and Soul and began to network with others in the HIV sector. When I was sure I was doing well on the treatment and felt fit enough

---

1   A CD4 count reveals how many disease-fighting T-cells are in your immune system. A normal healthy person's count would roughly be between 500 and 1500 per cubic millimetre of blood.

to work, I found a job with a small agency evaluating HIV projects. By this time, I had identified a void, since not many African people were speaking up about HIV, especially women. That was to be my mission and I haven't shut up talking about HIV since! I saw it as my role to support others living with HIV, especially those in the black African community, to persuade them they should seek testing and treatment. Many were reluctant for all sorts of reasons, for fear of side effects of the medication or that it would reveal to others they were HIV positive. Yet they were one of the groups most impacted by the virus, and if a husband failed to get tested or treated, he would risk passing it on to his wife and, through her, to future children.

We have to see HIV and AIDS as not just a local issue but a global one, which is why I began working in the international sector. How much stigma is attached to the virus, and how easy it is to access treatment, varies across the globe. There is still so much ignorance. In Africa, many people still lose their jobs and their livelihoods when they are found to be HIV positive. Through my international work on the issue, I visit many countries in sub-Saharan Africa where women and children living with HIV still have no access to treatment, because their governments can't afford to institute proper health care for them. There are also many widows and orphans who need support and aren't getting it. In Uganda, I co-founded a project supporting vulnerable young people so, before going to school, they can have breakfast: a cup of porridge with vitamins in it which helps them stay healthy and concentrate on lessons.

"I want everyone throughout the world to under-stand that people with HIV can live a full life and succeed in whatever they want to do ..."

Here I am, more than thirty years on, living a near-normal life in spite of the fact there is no cure. I want everyone throughout the world to understand that people with HIV can live a full life and succeed in whatever they want to do, without fear or prejudice. That's my way of paying back this precious gift of life I can now enjoy through HIV treatment.

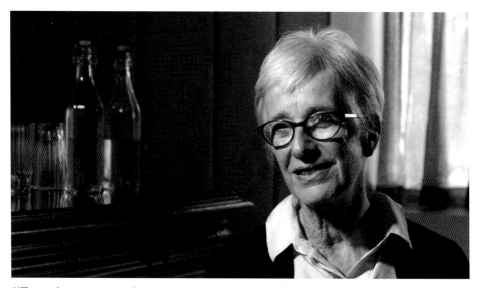

"In those early years, it was about partnership, that there were two of us feeling our way through this illness, doctor and patient."

Jane Anderson is a consultant physician who also chairs the National AIDS Trust, set up 30 years ago, which works to stop HIV from standing in the way of health, dignity and equality, and to end new HIV infections. She trained at St Mary's Hospital Medical School, qualifying in 1984. Her first job as a doctor was at St Mary's Hospital, working for the Professor of Medicine and for the Immunology team who oversaw the AIDS ward there. She went on to become a consultant at Barts Hospital and is now Director of the Homerton University Hospital NHS Foundation Trust Centre for the Study of Sexual Health and HIV.

"Our real challenge for the next decade, especially in the wake of Covid-19, will be ensuring that HIV remains a key priority …"

In the 1980s, doctors caring for people with AIDS faced a daunting task. They had to support and care for their patients through multiple, complex illnesses which were ultimately fatal without effective treatments for the virus; and some faced fear and prejudice from their own colleagues who were afraid of 'catching' HIV. Jane Anderson talks about the challenges she faced from her first day as a junior doctor, and throughout her career as a physician specialising in HIV and AIDS.

Professor Jane Anderson
"Dying before our eyes…"

On my first day as a newly qualified doctor in 1984, working at St Mary's, I was called to the AIDS ward to set up a drip for a very sick young man who was going blind from cytomegalovirus retinitis. In those days there was very little we could offer in the way of treatment for people with AIDS but, in this instance, huge vials of immunoglobulin had been flown in with the hope an infusion might help him. I was inexperienced and, try as I might, I could not get the cannula into his arm. So I rang an colleague to ask for help. When it was clear which ward I was on, it was suggested I call another colleague instead. Looking back, I think that moment shaped the rest of my career. I was shocked that a doctor would decline to help desperately sick patients, dying before our eyes.

In those days the AIDS ward at St Mary's was very unlike today's hospital wards. There were ten or twelve rooms, all single occupancy, painted a stark clinical cream. There was a set of cold, pretty bleak waiting areas in the corridor for visitors, and there was one huge room for the nursing staff and doctors, part medical hub, part social centre, warm and always full of cigarette smoke because in those days everyone smoked.

Barrier nursing was the order of the day, gloves, aprons and masks for the staff, not just because of the virus itself but because of other pathogens. People with AIDS could have a wide range of infectious conditions. Some patients were coughing with tuberculosis, others might have torrential diarrhoea. Everyone carries a whole variety

> "I was shocked that a doctor would decline to help desperately sick patients, dying before our eyes."

33

"Sometimes it was as if AIDS had an unnerving ability to target whatever was most precious."

of bacteria and pathogens they've met in the course of their life, which normally don't cause any bother so long as their immune system is strong. But the immune system needs only to weaken a little for TB to develop, so that would often be one of the early illnesses patients would present with, or perhaps shingles, depending on what they had encountered earlier in life. The more immunosuppressed they became, other bacteria or viruses they had been playing host to would get their chance. Pneumocystis, a fungus that causes pneumonia, tended to appear before cytomegalovirus. But being sick with pneumocystis would suppress the immune system further, so another condition would emerge. It also depended on where people had grown up. In parts of Africa, for instance, there's a strong link between HIV and TB, because so many people in Africa have already encountered the tuberculosis bacteria. Sometimes it was as if AIDS had an unnerving ability to target whatever was most precious. I cared for several visual artists who developed CMV retinitis and began to lose their sight.

There were difficult conversations with families, some learning for the first time their son was gay at the same time they had to grapple with knowing he had a fatal disease. Some refused to visit. And there was ongoing fear among a small minority of staff. We had to argue hard to get lab tests processed, if they required blood to be pipetted or handled manually. Even in 1990, when I set up the HIV unit at Bart's, there was a reluctance among some lab staff to process liver function tests. I had to explain that HIV positive blood was almost certainly going through their machines every day, from people in the community who hadn't been tested. All blood needed to be treated the same, because it was the specimen you *didn't* know about that was more dangerous.

"On the wards, though, the staff were utterly dedicated, even in the face of all the deaths."

On the wards, though, the staff were utterly dedicated, even in the face of all the deaths. In those early years, one of the most important aspects of our work was taking care of people – there was no magic pill. I went to a lot of funerals.

At first, in London, we were only seeing gay men with

AIDS. The first woman I saw with AIDS was from an African background. That was the point at which I realised AIDS was even more complicated than I'd originally assumed. Other questions began to emerge. What if a woman were pregnant? Could she or should she safely have children? This was the beginning of a new set of issues we needed to address though, of course, in some areas of Africa doctors were already seeing heterosexual people with HIV.

As doctors, the experience we were gaining with the illness meant that our careers moved more rapidly than we would have expected, as the number of posts were expanded in response to the epidemic. I went from being a junior houseman to consultant in just six years, appointed in 1990 to set up a new HIV unit at St Bartholomew's Hospital. Fortunately, we had powerful peer support and good networks – if a colleague didn't know the answer to your question, they might know somebody in New York or San Francisco who had experience of whatever it was.

By the time I became a registrar in 1987, the first antiretroviral drug, AZT, had been approved. At that time, it would normally take eight to ten years to get a drug fully trialled and approved. With AZT, the process took a matter of months, such was the need to find something that could stop the virus in its tracks. At the beginning there was a lack of understanding about how best to use it. Patients were given high doses every four hours. We issued them with pillboxes that had timers and beepers to wake them in the middle of the night to take their scheduled dose. And the side effects could be brutal. It often made patients anaemic, so they had to come into hospital for blood transfusions. Next came DDI, in big boxes of powder that needed to be mixed with water, tasting revolting. All the early drugs were unpleasant, some leaving people with a metallic taste in their mouth that never seemed to disappear. With the early protease inhibitors, the bioavailability – the proportion of the amount swallowed which can get from the gut into the bloodstream – was quite low, so that meant the quantity of tablets people had to take was enormous. Some patients

> "Other questions began to emerge. What if a woman were pregnant? Could she or should she safely have children?"

> "The first drug, AZT, had been approved. … And the side effects could be brutal."

> "Fortunately, by the early 1990s, other drugs were coming through and we used them more effectively."

> "Today's challenges are very different. The real shift has been that we are now aiming to test routinely people for HIV…"

were taking 18 pills, twice a day. We discovered that drinking grapefruit juice could block the enzymes in the liver that broke down the drug, so we recommended that. But still we weren't going fast enough developing new treatments that would save everyone. There was a real push and pull between activists and researchers to get the drugs approved faster – moving out of the labs and into sick people.

In those early years, it was about partnership, that there were two of us feeling our way through this illness, doctor and patient. Since we had only a few blunt instruments that still could not completely halt the disease in its tracks, it was essential that patients be involved in all decisions about what would allow them the best quality of life, whether to proceed with what were often punishing drug regimes – or not. New treatment information was shared – every few weeks pages of shiny fax paper would roll off the ward's machines – it was called Dr Fax – with information the activist community thought could be useful for us to know about.

Inevitably, when you start to challenge a virus, it fights back and is able to mutate, which can make it drug-resistant. Fortunately, by the early 1990s, other drugs were coming through and we used them more effectively. Once the structure of the virus became known, it was possible to make more targeted compounds designed to fit just one specific part of the virus, with new technologies in drug design being pioneered. HIV pushed the barriers in terms of biotechnology, in ways of measuring viruses and unpicking their genetic material to identify mutations. And as a result, our work as doctors now became much more technical. The power dynamic shifted, and the nature of partnership working between doctor and patient changed.

Today's challenges are very different. The real shift has been that we are now aiming to test people routinely for HIV in areas where it is most prevalent, whenever they come into contact with a health care professional, because the quicker people with the virus are able to access treatment, the better chance they have of staying well and living a long life and are not infectious to other people. And apart from anything else, this helps save the NHS money. We recommend anyone who is changing sexual partners regularly to take a test at least every three months, to help break the chain of transmission.

Looking to the future, Jonathan Mann was right in 1987 when he said we really need to see this as three separate but intertwined epidemics: AIDS, which we have largely been able to deal with; HIV, which increasingly we can solve; and finally, the social and political context, the way we plan for the future. We have effective treatments for the virus. But do we yet have social policies and a national strategy for the longer term consequences from this infection? People in Western Europe have lost a sense of the seriousness of HIV. They seem to think the epidemic is now over. But HIV and AIDS have not gone away. In fact, there are more people today living with HIV in this country than there have ever been. Our real challenge for the next decade, especially in the wake of Covid-19, will be ensuring that HIV remains a key priority – in order to end new infections and ensure that people living with HIV live long and live well.

"We have effective treatments for the virus. But do we yet have social policies and a national strategy for the longer term consequences from this infection?"

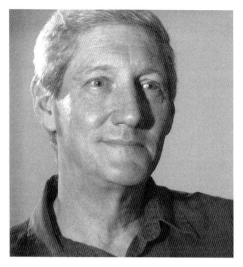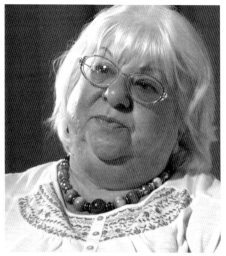

"There was, surprisingly, a lot of laughter. We all felt we were in it together."

After studying International Relations at Keele University, Sir Nick Partridge was living in Amsterdam when news of an illness affecting gay men in America started to percolate through to Europe. He returned to England, volunteered for Gay Switchboard, and then in 1985 secured a job as office administrator with the Terrence Higgins Trust (THT), the first charity in the UK to be set up in response to the AIDS pandemic. He went on to become its Chief Executive from 1991 to 2013. Honoured with an OBE in 1999 for his services to charity and knighted in 2009, he was named by the *Independent* in 2010 as one of the top 100 most influential gay and lesbian people in Britain.

Having graduated with a degree in social sciences and having qualified in social work in 1981, Janet Green was a volunteer on London Lesbian Line before starting at the Terrence Higgins Trust at the same time as Nick Partridge, sharing an office with him as the charity's first two paid employees. In her role as Counselling Co-ordinator, she was for the next eight years instrumental in setting up many of the charity's counselling and befriending initiatives. Afterwards, she continued to specialise in HIV as a local authority social worker, later working more generally in disability services, until her retirement in 2007.

From their different perspectives, Nick and Janet look back at the early years of the Terrence Higgins Trust and the support it offered to those with HIV and AIDS.

38

Sir Nick Partridge & Janet Green
"All in it together…"

NICK: My father told me it would be a mistake to apply for a job with the Terrence Higgins Trust as, once it was on my CV, it would blight my future career. I went ahead anyway. By then, there was a clear sense of foreboding among gay men in Europe. The number of people diagnosed in the US was doubling every six months and, to use Larry Kramer's words, the body count was rising. There was controversy still about how HIV was transmitted. Could you catch it through kissing? Through oral sex? Through mosquito bites? Through a simple touch? We were quite rightly fearful of a new infectious disease and outraged that governments around the world were ignoring it. Society split between those who saw the need for care and compassion and those who wanted to distance themselves and ostracise people with HIV. I knew which camp I wanted to be in.

"It was a steep learning curve …"

At the start the Terrence Higgins Trust, like Gay Switchboard, was wholly volunteer-run. Terry Higgins was one of the first men in the UK to die with AIDS and it had been founded in his name by his lover and friends.[1] Most of the people involved were volunteers in their twenties and thirties and had scant understanding of how to work with health services, social services, local and central government, how to raise money, how to apply for grants or even how to become a charity. It was a steep learning curve. When Gay Switchboard had applied for charitable status a few years earlier, the charity commissioners rejected their application on the basis that, in their view, the provision of support and information to homosexuals was not an appropriate charitable activity. THT learned from that and, when it applied for charitable status in 1983, instead of emphasising the gay community, it hinged the application on its support for people with AIDS.

---

[1] Rupert Whitaker (see later in book), Tony Calvert, Martyn Butler, Len Robinson and Chris Peel, later joined by Tony Whitehead who became the first chair of its steering committee.

JANET: Until the 1980s, gay men and lesbians rarely mixed. They had their bars, we had ours. We even had separate Pride marches. I remember a colleague on the London Lesbian Line saying to me: "Why on earth would you want to go and work with gay men?" But there had been a time in my life when gay men had been very kind to me and, although what I knew about the scientific side of HIV and AIDS would barely have covered the back of a postage stamp, I was becoming increasingly concerned and angry about the media coverage. Young men were getting ill and dying and being reviled by the tabloids. One newspaper campaign suggested everyone with HIV should be dumped on the Isle of Wight in a kind of leper colony. I wanted to do something.

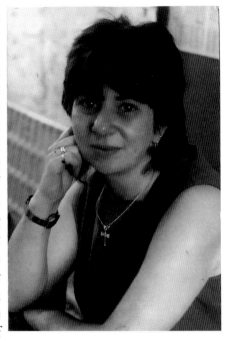

> "I was becoming increasingly concerned and angry about the media coverage."

During the job interview, I asked how many other women were involved in the Trust. There was a long pause and some shifty looks. "About ten," someone said. There were actually two, and that included me. But it soon changed.

That first day, there was Nick Partridge sitting across the desk from me. We smiled at each other and I think he was as bewildered and unprepared as I was. But we made it up as we went along – if it worked, great. If not, we tried something else.

The offices were in Clerkenwell and it was the most dilapidated, rundown building I've ever worked in, freezing in winter, boiling hot in summer, overcrowded. I was constantly having to shoo volunteers off my desk. I was working 12- or 14-hour days, it was emotionally tough and full-on, but I loved it. There was, surprisingly, a lot of laughter. We all felt we were in it together. There were no sharp dividing lines between volunteers and service users, and I found myself supporting both.

I started by developing training for the helpline. There was already a buddy[2] service, but it was in its infancy, with referrals which tended to be done on the back of a cigarette packet, so it needed to be organised and professionalised, especially as we soon began to gather more and more volunteers.

NICK: We may have lacked experience but we did have a blueprint. In the US, gay organisations had already pioneered the buddy system to support people abandoned by their families, and that became the living heart of THT. We shamelessly stole from the training manuals our American colleagues had devised, and assigned volunteers to local groups, each covering a different area in London. As soon as the call from a hospital came in, a suitable buddy volunteer would be briefed. Incredible friendships were created as a result.

There was very little money. A grant had been secured from the Greater London Council (GLC) under Ken Livingstone – Red Ken, the right-wing press called him – to fund my post and that of Janet Green, but the Conservative-run Westminster City Council led by Dame Shirley Porter took the GLC to court to prevent the money being paid[3]. We were saved by an astounding level of support from drag queens like Lily Savage, who put on benefits for us in pubs and clubs and, later, theatre people and musicians like Elton John. Without them, the charity would not have survived.

Soon we had the helpline, buddy group, health promotion group, a counselling group, a welfare rights group, a medical group whose task was to interpret the latest developments in scientific understanding of the virus, a legal group who fought cases of unfair dismissal, and an interfaith group which provided a space for gay men and women of faith to come together. It produced, for instance, a leaflet *Is The Chalice Safe?* setting out the facts of HIV transmission for

"As soon as the call from a hospital came in, a suitable buddy volunteer would be briefed. Incredible friendships were created as a result."

---

2 The 'buddies' close the gap between an HIV test and professional counselling services. Buddies do not offer classic professional advice but let others share their life experiences.

3 Ironically Westminster was to become one of the London boroughs most affected by AIDS.

people worried they might pass on or pick up the virus if they participated in Holy Communion. There were always arguments, egos, squabbles over funding and priorities, and sometimes the steering committee meetings went on long past midnight as people jockeyed to promote their particular corner, but it was an extraordinary blossoming of community activism.

We broke new ground in finding ways to get the message across about safe sex, knowing we would be listened to in a way a government campaign might not be. No gay men used condoms in 1980, but many, many did so by 1985. Our health promotion group provided leaflets promoting condom use and, as a side benefit, we saw a dramatic drop in cases of gonorrhoea, syphilis and other sexually transmitted infections. It's something we should always be immensely proud of as a community, because not only did we change risky sexual behaviours, we also started the country talking about sex in a way it had never done previously. There was a mistaken belief before AIDS that sex had become safe for the first time in human history, with the Pill to prevent pregnancy and antibiotics to cure most STIs. But now sex was dangerous again, and the only way to eliminate the danger was to talk about what goes on in the bedroom, gay or straight.

> "I've always loved the fact that THT never lost its sense of humour and was never anti-sex."

At that point, we began to realise how little we knew about the sex lives of gay men. If you are going to deliver effective health campaigns around sex or, indeed, drug use, you have to root those in evidence and prioritise the greatest risks. It caused huge and often hilarious rows in our meetings, because each thought his own sex life represented what the majority of gay men did. So we carried out surveys and asked people to keep diaries, to gain a better understanding of the wonderful diversity of gay men's sexual behaviour – how many were in long term couples, how many serially monogamous, and how many partied wildly with lots and lots of different partners – not nearly as many as you might imagine from press reports! I've always loved the fact that THT never lost its sense of humour and was never anti-sex.

JANET: In the wider community, there was a lot of fear. We were getting sackloads of letters from worried people who needed help. Unfortunately, there were also quite a few letters from bigots, written in green ink and capital letters, which went straight in the bin but were nonetheless upsetting.

We heard of patients in hospital whose meals were left outside the door of their room, of hospices that wouldn't take them, of undertakers who refused to bury them. One day we were having new office furniture delivered and, when the delivery men realised who we were, they refused to come in and left our new chairs on the pavement in the rain.

Insurance companies wouldn't insure anyone who took a test for HIV, even if they tested negative – simply getting tested, regardless of the result, was considered a verdict on your lifestyle and damned you. People with AIDS were excluded from some benefits such as Disability Living Allowance or Attendance Allowance. Even though they would be dead soon, it was felt they weren't ill enough. One man I knew cunningly dropped a tab of acid just before his assessment and behaved so bizarrely it was concluded he had dementia and therefore qualified for a benefit.

> **"Insurance companies wouldn't insure anyone who took a test for HIV, even if they tested negative."**

At first, we were only seeing gay and bisexual men, though later there were some women, usually injecting drug users. In 1985, there was no treatment for the virus, and people understood that a diagnosis meant they were going to die. Some seemed to lose the will to live and died quite quickly after being diagnosed. Others said, "Stuff this, I'm fighting back."

A volunteer, Jim Wilson, was one such. When people called for help, I would sometimes say: "Would you like to meet someone who's already been diagnosed?" And Jim would travel right across London at the drop of a hat. He identified the need to do something for men with HIV in prison and set up a prison visiting service. He was into his leathers, had the moustache, a 'clone' as many gay men were at the time, tall, thin, dark and incredibly handsome. But he was also funny and feisty and had a strong sensitive side. I heard about one meeting of volunteers where there was a woman in the room; some of the gay men didn't like it and were being bitchy. But Jim said: "Are you completely stupid? Because when we get ill, who's going to be left to look after us? It's going to be our women friends." Much as I tried to keep a professional distance, some people I met there did touch me emotionally and Jim, who became a close friend, was one of them. I was devastated when he died.

> **"AIDS brought together gay and lesbian communities in a way not seen previously."**

NICK: AIDS brought together gay and lesbian communities in a way not seen previously. You have to remember that gay men and women had very different histories and there'd been few places where their interests were seen to coincide – indeed there was an element of traditional misogyny among some older gay men. But so great was this crisis that lesbians saw gay men needed help, as did many sympathetic straight people, and came forward. All of us, I think, were afraid AIDS might be used as an excuse to roll back the small advances in equality we'd gained, which helped forge the alliance between lesbians and gay men.[4]

As a result, we were able to build on what had been learned from the feminist health movement in the 1970s, which aimed to de-medicalise services like maternity care and gynaecology and make them more responsive to women's needs. The best of the doctors and nurses we dealt with understood immediately that, without listening to what people with AIDS were saying, it would be much harder to come up with treatments or care that worked.

We were also fortunate that, although the Department of Health was determined not to be seen as kowtowing to a bunch of gay men, the Chief Medical Officer at the time, Donald Acheson, was an epidemiologist and sympathetic. He gave me his private telephone number and told me to call him at home, so civil servants in the department couldn't listen in. We also had a sympathetic response from the Secretary of State of Health, Norman Fowler, who set up a separate Cabinet committee on HIV to take decision-making away from the cabinet as a whole, and the baleful influence of Margaret Thatcher. [5]

There were those in the gay community who thought we'd lost our radical edge and shouldn't be cosying up to the Establishment but, to be effective bringing about change, you can't remain on the outside lobbing hand grenades in. If you are to have a long term, determined and effective response, you have to occupy some of the central ground, to win the respect of decision makers in government and the professions.

"… some were cared for lovingly by parents and siblings, others were completely abandoned, by friends as well as family."

JANET: I felt so sorry for the younger gay men who were angry and despondent and wanted their mums – though they couldn't always call on their mothers for support. Though some were cared for lovingly by parents

---

4   A fear crystallised later, in 1988, by Section 28 of the Local Government Act which sought to prevent the "promotion of homosexuality by local authorities and in schools."
5   Lord Fowler went on to become a Patron of the Terrence Higgins Trust, and has also contributed an essay to this book.

and siblings, others were completely abandoned, by friends as well as family. Many faced the dilemma of coming out to their families as a gay man at the same time they had to reveal they had HIV or AIDS. And though that was always heart-wrenching, sometimes it could be humorous. One lad went home to his parents for the weekend to break the news. There was a sharp intake of breath, until his father, obviously completely flummoxed, came out with: "Son, the world has just fallen out of your mother's bottom." Whether his parents managed to laugh when they realised how Dad had muddled the words, I have no idea, but we howled about it in the office.

NICK: As we grew as an organisation and became more professional, some of that initial improvisatory spirit had to fall by the wayside. There were clashes: it's heart-breaking to have to agree a policy on the number of funerals staff can attend in paid time, or deal with disgruntled volunteers when unions quite sensibly insisted we institute a no-smoking policy in our new building: "We're giving you our time and now you say we can't smoke. It's AIDS killing us, not the odd cigarette in the office."

But the commitment of both staff and volunteers was extraordinary, a life-affirming response to the cruel and hostile circumstances in which we found ourselves. Funerals became celebrations of life, where the instruction was to wear something bright, not black. Funerals with glitter balls. Funerals where the coffin slid through the curtains accompanied by a joyous disco track. I like to think we played a part in changing the way many funerals are now conducted in the UK. The wakes were amazing, though new dilemmas emerged – what's the etiquette of cruising at a funeral?

JANET: When I had to leave THT, made redun-

> "But the commitment of staff and volunteers was extraordinary, a life-affirming response in the cruel and hostile circumstances in which we found ourselves."

dant as a result of a funding crisis in 1993 – ironically only shortly before Freddie Mercury died and left the charity a large bequest – I was heartbroken. I continued to work in HIV services for a local authority, where I was dealing with many more women now, many of them immigrants from sub-Saharan Africa whose plight was desperate.

"Together, we managed to change the public understanding of what it means to be gay, and build the case for equality …"

NICK: The lowest point was, for me, 1993. As well as funding difficulties, the results of the first international clinical trial into the efficacy of AZT, the main treatment at the time, were really disappointing. The numbers dying, and the numbers diagnosed each year, were increasing. You couldn't travel to the US if you had HIV.[6] Everything seemed to be going the wrong way. Yet still we soldiered on.

Little did I know that less than three years away was a real breakthrough in terms of treatment, one that would completely reverse the curve. The only sadness was that it would come too late for so many. Now I know that we helped bring that about. Between 1983 and the late 1990s, close to 300 charities were set up in the UK with HIV and AIDS as the core of their work, offering a real diversity of service provision. Together, we managed to change the public understanding of what it means to be gay, and build the case for equality – and if you'd told me in 1985 that, one day, I'd be able to marry my long-term partner, Simon, I'd have thought you a lunatic. We should be immensely proud of all that we achieved.

---

6   Jim Wilson was discovered with AZT in his luggage when he flew into Philadelphia and was put on the next plane back.

JANET: Looking back at the legacy of that time, it was the beginning of a different sort of gay community. Gay men have always had women friends, but we came together in a different way, with more and more lesbians becoming buddies at THT or volunteering on the helpline. There was a feeling that these were our people, and we were all in it together. Such strong friendships were forged in those years, resulting in men and women standing shoulder to shoulder at Pride marches, and the widening of the movement to include all variations of sex and gender. I'm so grateful I was there and played a part.

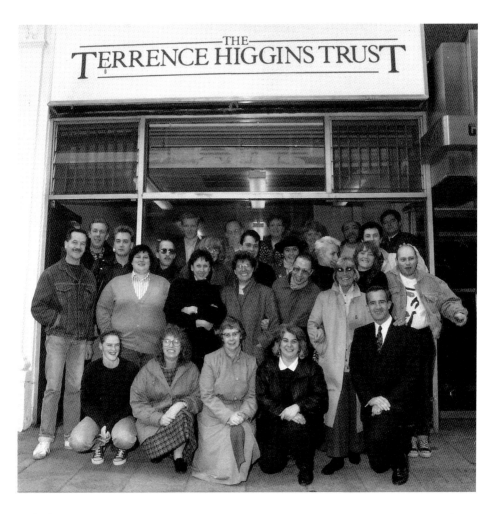

"There was a feeling that these were our people, and we were all in it together. Such strong friendships were forged in those years …"

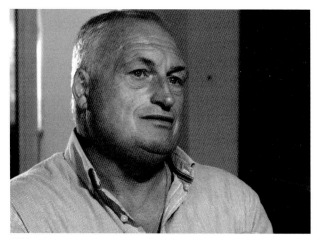

"I tried not to let haemophilia get in the way of anything I wanted to do…"

"Like a stone thrown into a pond, the ripples go out and the whole family suffers."

Alan Burgess was diagnosed as a child in 1967 with a moderate form of haemophilia. A painter and decorator by trade, he was married with children in the 1980s when he was given NHS contaminated blood products and became infected with HIV, eventually losing his business and much else besides. He joined the Birchgrove Support Group, a campaigning group set up by haemophiliacs with HIV, and has given evidence to the Infected Blood Inquiry which got underway in 2018.

"Our GP … told us to put our faith in God and pray everything would be all right."

Haemophilia is a genetically-transmitted inherited bleeding disorder that tends to affect males rather than females, caused by the lack of a clotting factor in the blood. It is usually diagnosed in childhood and those who have it are at risk of bleeding uncontrollably if they suffer an injury. In the 1960s, doctors began using cryoprecipitate, a by-product of frozen donated blood plasma and rich in the proteins that help clotting, to treat haemophiliacs. By the 1970s, a more convenient concentrated freeze-dried product, Factor VIII, derived from many thousands of pints of donated blood, was available. Unfortunately, some blood donors, especially in the US, were not being rigorously screened and, in the UK, the DOH were sending teams to prisons and borstals to harvest blood from inmates. As a result Factor VIII was dangerously contaminated with HIV and hepatitis B and C. So, as a consequence of commercial providers and the NHS using this blood, many haemophiliacs were infected and, even after the scandal was revealed, have received no compensation, just small piecemeal, ex-gratia payments.

Alan Burgess
"We didn't dare tell anyone."

As a haemophiliac, I always had to be careful. If I so much as bumped against something, I might start bleeding internally into a joint, which would become painful and inflamed and, unless the bleed could be stopped, the joint suffered lifelong damage. I tried not to let haemophilia get in the way of anything I wanted to do, so I used to lead a fairly active life. In 1982, I got a knock playing football which led to me being treated with a contaminated batch of NHS Factor VIII at Addenbrooke's Hospital in Cambridge.

Three years later, in 1985, my haematologist phoned me to say haemophiliacs in the UK were being routinely tested for what was then called HTLV-3, later to be called HIV, after some in the US had become infected – but there was nothing to worry about, as British blood products were thought to be safe. I was tested, thought no more of it, but a few weeks later a brown envelope turned up in the post. And that was how I found out I had tested positive for the AIDS virus – by letter.

My wife and I made an appointment to see the haematologist in my local hospital. She was utterly useless, didn't have a clue. She said: "You know, you might be lucky. Not everybody dies with it." I thought: *Die?* How can I die at 28?

"You know, you might be lucky. Not everybody dies with it."

We were so confused we made an appointment to see a haematologist at the hospital where I'd received Factor VIII, but she was even less help. She implied we were wasting her time, as we'd already seen the haematologist in Suffolk. She was so dismissive of our plight my wife started to cry and was upset but we didn't get any advice about how to live with the virus.

Within two months, my wife was pregnant with our third child, and it was only then we realised what we were facing. After having no joy in trying to find advice on whether to have the pregnancy terminated, our GP was our last port of call. He told us that, as far as he knew, both my wife and baby could be infected. Again, the advice he gave us was hardly practical. He told us to put our faith in God and pray everything would be all right. When Denise went into labour, she was put in a room on her own at the bottom of a long corridor in the maternity unit, with yellow biohazard stickers both on the door and in the room. We were both warned not to tell anyone of my status in the maternity ward as it would lead to patients discharging themselves along with the new-born babies, such was the fear of AIDS at the time. Fortunately, both she and the baby tested negative.

We were advised not to tell anyone. And lived our lives accordingly. One day I was painting the next-door neighbour's house with one of the men who worked for me, and my wife was in our garden hanging out the washing. The radio was on, and a news item came on about Rock Hudson dying of AIDS. "Know what I'd do?" said my workmate. "Line 'em up against a wall and shoot the bloody lot of 'em. Dirty bastards" Denise heard him and shouted: "You have that attitude and you won't be working for my husband!" though I was frantically trying to shut her up in case it made him suspicious.

"Suddenly I realised I wasn't alone …"

At this stage I hadn't been referred to an AIDS specialist. It was two years before I became ill. I kept getting serious chest infections but, being self-employed, I'd struggle back to work as soon as I could – there's no sick pay when you work for yourself. Believe it or not, at that time I'd never even met another haemophiliac – there aren't many out in the sticks in Suffolk. But I heard the Haemophilia Society was planning a class legal action, so I got in touch and went to a meeting in Newcastle. Suddenly I realised I wasn't alone, and that the treatment I'd been getting was shockingly inadequate. Afterwards I stormed into my haematologist's office and was finally referred to a chest specialist.

It was six years before the NHS let slip that I'd also been infected with Hepatitis C, and that I'm at risk of CJD – Creutzfeldt-Jakob, mad cow disease – from NHS contaminated blood products.

As haemophiliacs, we could see the gay community organising a social support network and how strong it was, so we started a support group called the Birchgrove. The people I met there were like brothers, the only ones who could really understand how I felt, and some of those friendships have lasted to this day. When the first treatments arrived, I was placed on AZT, but the side effects were horrendous, I'd never had headaches like it, I was nauseous, and had stomach problems along with acute diarrhoea which led to one of many hospital stays at the time. I dreaded putting those tablets in my mouth. By now my poor health had dictated that I'd had to give up work, because the doctor told me that if I didn't, I'd be dead within six months. If I stopped work, she added, I possibly had two years left. Unfortunately AZT wasn't the only AIDS drug I had to endure. Over the following years a toxic cocktail of drugs, again with horrendous side effects were given in an attempt to keep me alive. Some of the long-term effects of those drugs I am suffering now and will do for the rest of my life.

In 1988, the government set up the McFarlane Trust to give us £20,000 each as a one-off payment. I suspect they saw it as a quick solution to a short-term problem, because we'd all be dead within two or three years. But we saw it as an admission of guilt and pressed on with the class action. Under John Major's government in 1991, we were told we were to get a larger payment as an out-of-court settlement, but were told by our solicitors that everyone had to agree to the amount or it would be withdrawn. Another condition was that we had to sign a waiver saying we promised no further legal action over blood-borne viruses. I'd just been told I only had two years to live, so I'd lost the will to fight and I signed. But evidence presented to the current Inquiry has shown that the government were aware and knew that all the haemophiliacs infected with HIV also had Hepatitis C thus morally blackmailing us into signing the waiver which to this day shows how corrupt and dishonest governments can be.

We told the children when they were old enough to understand and, as a family, withdrew into ourselves. But people locally were beginning to get suspicious of what was wrong with me and put two and two together. Denise was grilled by other parents when she did the school run: "Why's your Alan ill again?" Whispers went round; our car was vandalised. The children were having a bad time at school, with some other children being nasty. One of my daughters went without school dinners because she dreaded standing in the queue for free school dinners as she thought it was shameful, and other kids would mock her and the family for having free school dinners. We had problems later with

> "… we started a support group called the Birchgrove. The people I met there were like brothers, the only ones who could really understand how I felt, and some of those friendships have lasted to this day."

> "Staying alive was gruelling, and I was angry this had been done to me. The trouble with anger is you take it out on those around you."

her during her teenage years, when she self-harmed. I only recently understood it was because she was under such stress, believing I was going to die, and found my prolonged bouts of illness and hospital stays harrowing. Like a stone thrown into a pond, the ripples go out and the whole family suffers.

We lived in a small close and some people had stopped talking to us. The house was vandalised while we were on holiday. With that, along with damage to the car, we felt we had no option but to move. However, because of my HIV, we couldn't get life insurance or a normal mortgage, and were lucky eventually to get an interest-only one. But without life insurance, or mortgage protection. I had to build up savings to be able eventually to pay off the principal, and that got me into trouble with the Department of Work and Pensions who wanted to remove my benefits because I was over the savings threshold and over the years we had many demoralising visits from officials from DWP going through every aspect of our finances which stripped even more layers of dignity from both me and my wife.

Mentally, I was falling apart. I felt unclean and that I shouldn't go near my wife in case I infected her. Our sex life, which used to be brilliant, went right out of the window. My business had gone to the wall and we'd have lost the house if it hadn't been for the money from the government. Staying alive was gruelling, and I was angry this had been done to me. The trouble with anger is you take it out on those around you. After a row at home, I'd get in the car and stay out all night. Friends from the Birchgrove Group were dying, and I attended many funerals. I felt so depressed that I began to think I should be dead too and planned to commit suicide, but was found in time and committed to a psychiatric hospital. Although I came out after a month feeling better, the depression hung over me and I wasn't very nice to live with so Denise and I eventually split up, and I sofa-surfed at my sister's and other places until an AIDS social worker helped me find a place of my own. Even that was a fight – the council wanted to put me in a bedsit, although I needed a spare room for my daughters who would come and care for me when I was ill, and for the nebuliser I needed to prevent my pneumocystis pneumonia (PCP) recurring.

When I was finally alone in my new abode, I took stock of my life and realised I couldn't carry on like I was. My AIDS social worker managed to get me counselling, although just to visit the counsellor it meant a round trip of 100 miles, such was the shortage of qualified AIDS counsellors. After three long

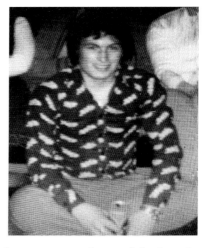

years, I'm glad to say eventually Denise and I got back together, although to this day I still suffer from depression. In fact, my doctor said I probably had Post Traumatic Stress Syndrome. When he said that, my retort was "POST? There's nothing POST about my stress; I will have the stress of what happened to me and AIDS until the day I die!" But I have learned to live with things, I now cope in a better way and I chose to be open about having HIV and I gave an interview to a Sunday newspaper and interviews to the TV. Just to prove stigma towards those of us with AIDS hasn't gone away, the week before the newspaper article was published, the window cleaner came round and saw all my HIV medication laid out on the table as Denise was busy putting them into Dossett boxes. He asked who was ill, and Denise decided she might as well tell him about my condition, as it was going to be in the paper. That was the last time we saw that window cleaner, though he still does the neighbours' windows!

Did we ever get justice? Over the years we squeezed a bit more money out of the government, after they started yet another begging scheme for us, but we are still awaiting proper compensation, something we are hoping that the present Public Inquiry addresses when it eventually reports. But yet more of us will have died due to long-term co-morbidities, suffering from, amongst other things, coronary vascular disease, kidney disease, liver problems, cancer and joint problems – brought on, we believe, by being long-term AIDS survivors. As for justice, we're still waiting for the Infected Blood Inquiry, which got underway in 2018, to establish the basis for some form of redress, but it will never bring back the 1,100 haemophiliacs that were cruelly robbed of their lives. Originally there were 1,243 haemophiliacs infected with HIV in the UK. Now there are fewer than 250 or so of us left. HIV casts a long shadow.

I have no idea why I'm still alive, when so many just like me have died, as this awful disease seems to have no logical explanation as to who is taken and who is spared. One thing I am sure of though is that I couldn't have survived if it wasn't for the love and support of my wife Denise and daughters Sarah and Laura. For that I will be eternally grateful.

"I couldn't have survived if it wasn't for the love and support of my wife and daughters."

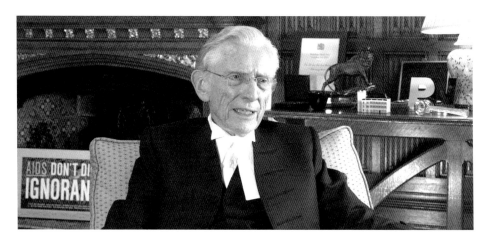

"These stories need to be told, because it is all too easy to forget. I would hope that people in future will be able to learn from them and make better decisions as a result."

After a career in journalism, Norman Fowler was elected as a Conservative Member of Parliament in 1970. He served in Margaret Thatcher's government in the 1980s, first as Minister of Transport and then as Secretary of State for Health and Social Security, remaining in that post from 1981 to 1987 and overseeing the government's response to HIV and AIDS, including the memorable advertising campaign to raise awareness in 1987. He then became Employment Secretary but resigned from the Cabinet in 1990. He was knighted in the same year. Later he returned to frontline politics as Chairman of the Conservative Party from 1992–94, then sat on the Conservative front bench from 1997 to 1999 as a member of the Shadow Cabinet, finally stepping down as an MP in 2001. He became a Conservative life peer, Baron Fowler of Sutton Coldfield, and entered the House of Lords. Renouncing party political allegiance, he became Lord Speaker in 2016, a post he held until April 2021. He continues to campaign for LGBT rights and to raise awareness of HIV and AIDS as an UNAIDS ambassador and is a Patron of the Terrence Higgins Trust.

As Minister of Health in the mid-1980s, Lord Fowler found himself at odds with Margaret Thatcher and other members of the Cabinet over how much attention should be paid to the AIDS pandemic. Some neat political manoeuvring enabled him to run a memorable public health campaign which made the nation aware that HIV and AIDS could affect anyone.

Lord Fowler
"Don't Die of Ignorance."

When the question of how to deal with AIDS in the UK arose in the mid-1980s, it seemed to me there were very few policy options. We could have ignored it, and there were plenty of people in government saying just that. I had little connection with either the LGBT community or drug users, among whom the disease was spreading fastest, but I could not understand the arguments of those who said it was nothing to do with us. As Health Secretary, I felt we had a duty to get the message out to as many people as possible that this was a terrible condition and a public health issue. There was no vaccine and there was no cure.

The man who did most to bring it home to me was Donald Acheson, who was the Chief Medical Officer. If Donald said this was a serious issue and likely to worsen, you could be sure he was right. He predicted that if infection rates continued to rise, within a couple of years there would be 20,000 people with HIV in the UK – which then meant 20,000 deaths.

There were some who believed this was not a public health issue but one of public morality. The Chief Rabbi was one of the most vociferous, telling me my policy should be to say plainly that AIDS was the consequence of sexual deviation, marital infidelity, social irresponsibility and a generation who put pleasure before duty and discipline. Frankly, my view was that if a government is so foolish as to run a moral campaign, the first time a Minister is caught with their pants down or putting cocaine up their nose, the

> "There were some who believed this was not a public health issue but one of public morality."

"…we wanted to try something similar to combat high rates of HIV among injecting drug users, by distributing clean needles to addicts. … I ran into serious opposition."

whole campaign goes up in smoke. I was proved right a few years later when John Major's *Back to Basics* campaign, an appeal for a return to traditional values, was ridiculed after a series of scandals involving Conservative politicians.

Our only weapon to fight the disease was publicity, and I was determined to get a strong campaign going – "Don't die of ignorance" – with a leaflet sent to every household in the country. But Margaret Thatcher, though she showed a good appreciation of the science when I took Donald Acheson to brief her, was convinced I was becoming obsessed: "Norman," she said, "you mustn't just be known as the Minister for AIDS." I thought for a moment that might mean I would next be promoted to Chancellor of the Exchequer, but no such luck. The subtext was: Norman, you're spending far too much time on this subject, kindly go and do something else. Though she might not have put it in quite the same terms as the Chief Rabbi, her view was in some respects very similar: if we gave out explicit information about what kinds of sexual activity were risky, we could expose young people to the shock of knowing things they would be much better off not knowing.

The way I always handled Margaret was that, if there was likely to be a point of conflict, it was safest to go round her, rather than through her. I had a number of opponents in the Cabinet as a whole, so getting agreement on anything was time-consuming and difficult. Lord Hailsham, a grand old man of politics, criticised me for the phrase 'having sex' in one of our advertisements. "Quite inappropriate," he huffed. "Is there no limit to vulgarity?"

Robert Armstrong, the Cabinet Secretary, Ken Stowe, my Permanent Secretary in the DHSS, and Donald Acheson hatched a plan with me to set up a separate committee within Cabinet to hammer out policy for AIDS and HIV. To my great relief, the efficient and broadly sympathetic William Whitelaw was appointed to chair it – I'd recently had an exhausting experience trying to get policy through a Cabinet committee on Social Security with Margaret in the chair. We managed to ensure neither Lord Hailsham nor Norman Tebbit, another fierce opponent of AIDS policy, were on the committee.

The leaflet was quickly endorsed by the committee, as were most of the proposals we discussed, though by no means all. Donald was an advocate of practical health initiatives. His great-grandfather was a medical man at the time of the First World War. There was a terrible problem of venereal disease among the troops. A campaign was run: "Think of Queen and Country." Hardly surprisingly, it had little effect. Only when someone had the bright idea of issuing the troops with the forerunner to condoms did the incidence of VD began to fall. It was a lovely example of practical public health policy and we wanted to try something similar to combat high rates of HIV among injecting drug users, by distributing clean needles to addicts. But though I had the backing of almost every independent committee that looked at the issue, I ran into serious opposition. The view was that giving out free needles effectively condoned crime, whereas I felt that was hardly the issue: we should not leave drug users to continue sharing dirty needles. After a great deal of argument, it was approved, but I am convinced that if William Whitelaw had put it to a vote, instead of simply summing up in our favour, we might well have lost.

The advertising campaign attracted a lot of criticism. It was accused of being overdramatic, with its tombstones and icebergs and John Hurt's marvellous voice-over, but I make no apologies. We had tried discreet little paragraphs in the newspapers, to absolutely no effect whatsoever. If we were to have any impact at all we needed to wake people up. Fortunately, the committee agreed. We put up posters, we ran television and cinema commercials, aiming for language that was both forceful and

"If we were to have any impact at all we needed to wake people up. … The infection rate of HIV went down and, interestingly, so did the incidence of other sexually transmitted diseases."

"… getting agreement on anything was time-consuming and difficult …"

"… ask ourselves what future generations might say about us too. Will they ask why we allowed 36 million to die? Couldn't we have done something to prevent it? And, of course, we could."

scientifically accurate. Later we did a follow-up poll and over 90% of the public agreed with the way it was done. To be honest, I am not used as a politician to getting 90% support, so it felt like a vindication. The infection rate of HIV went down and, interestingly, so did the incidence of other sexually transmitted diseases.

In 1987, I flew to the United States to see if there was anything we could learn from them. But the Federal Government was doing very little, leaving it to state administrations, who weren't doing much either: any progress was achieved by activists in the gay community. I visited a hospital in San Francisco and was photographed shaking hands with a young man who had AIDS – this was some months before Princess Diana created a far greater stir by doing the same. When I returned, Margaret Thatcher and Norman Tebbit, the Party Chairman, were outraged a British Minister had been photographed meeting, as they thought, unsavoury characters. I suspect my successor at the Health Ministry, John Moore, was told in no uncertain terms he should concentrate on other matters and not follow in my footsteps.

A senior Cabinet minister said to me not so long ago: "Well, no one dies from AIDS anymore." That shows the lack of understanding among even intelligent people. Globally, we have now lost 36 million people to AIDS according to UNAIDS. I am somewhat sympathetic to people who knock down statues of slave owners because I think we should take a lesson from it and ask ourselves what future generations might say about us too. Will they ask why we allowed 36 million to die? Couldn't we have done something to prevent it? And, of course, we could. We could stand up against the prejudice against gay people and the stigma of HIV worldwide, especially in some parts of Africa and certain countries in

Eastern Europe. We could do more for the families of those who die and those who suffer an impoverished old age.

By far the most persuasive factor in removing stigma and the wall of silence that allows infections to go on rising, is for people to come out and say they are HIV+, telling us what it has been like for them. These stories need to be told, because it is all too easy to forget. I would hope that people in future will be able to learn from them and make better decisions as a result.

"We could stand up against the prejudice against gay people and the stigma of HIV worldwide, especially in some parts of Africa and certain countries in Eastern Europe. We could do more for the families of those who die and those who suffer an impoverished old age."

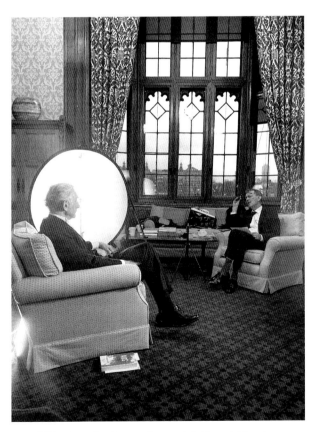

Filming the interview with Lord Fowler

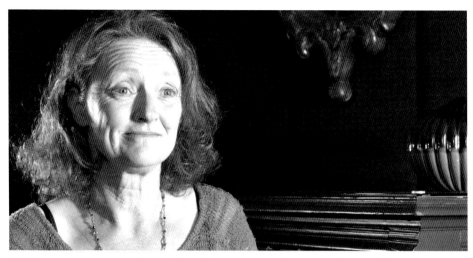

"I have never laughed so much as when I was with them, or cried as much."

Born into a theatrical family, Kelly Hunter made her debut on the London stage in 1979 at the age of 17, in the original production of the musical *Evita*. Over her career she has appeared in leading roles in musicals and joined the Royal Shakespeare Company and the National Theatre, as well as acting on television and in films. She began working with autistic children while she was at the RSC and founded Flute Theatre, her own theatre company, to bring Shakespeare to children who otherwise would have little access to the arts. She has developed her own technique, The Hunter Heartbeat Method, a series of sensory and communicative games based on the essence of Shakespeare for autistic people to play. As well as winning awards for her theatre and radio performances, she was awarded the MBE in 2019 for services to theatre.

"It was profoundly moving that a bunch of people, pilloried by society and told that AIDS was their own fault, were utterly non-judgmental themselves."

When Kelly Hunter's close friends in the theatre began dying of AIDS related illness, she put her career on hold for two years to volunteer with the Terrence Higgins Trust. She used her theatrical contacts to raise money for AIDS charities and was the driving force behind some of the most memorable fundraising initiatives of the late 1980s.

Kelly Hunter MBE
"I wanted to make a difference …"

I'd made a lot of gay friends in the theatre, and before long everyone began to hear whispers about AIDS and sense the beginning of fear, which only seemed to make some people party harder. Tuesday night was 'Straight Night' at the gay club Heaven, under the arches of the Embankment, so everyone from the West End shows, straight and gay, would head there after the curtain went down, and dance until dawn. But the nearer the illness came, the less easy it was to have conversations with people about it.

My closest gay friend was Geoffrey Burridge, an actor who was in *Emmerdale* and *Blake's Seven*, and the film *An American Werewolf in London*. He became very ill and I remember seeing the fear in his face. When he died, it was the most seismic event in my life. I was only 23 and I'd had some success in West End musicals – after *Evita*, I'd played Sally Bowles in *Cabaret* – but it meant nothing to me after Geoffrey's death. I felt I owed it to Geoffrey to put my career on hold, though my family told me I was making a terrible mistake, and give all my time to volunteering with the Terrence Higgins Trust. Doing that seemed so much more real than my life in the theatre.

On the top floor of the building in the Gray's Inn Road where the Trust had its offices, a self-help group for men with HIV, called Frontliners, was based. I grew to know them all well. Many were too ill to work and had difficulty getting benefits, but they were a lovely bunch of people, warm and funny, full of gallows humour – I have never laughed so much as when I was with them, or cried as much. Almost all were as camp as Chloe: they loved feather boas and played *It's Raining Men* all the time in the office. There was just one straight guy, an Irishman called John Maudaunt. He had been a heroin addict who picked up HIV through sharing needles and somehow blundered into THT in a state of panic, never having met a gay man in his life before. But I loved the way the gay men took him in as a brother and didn't judge him at all for his lifestyle. It was profoundly moving that a bunch of people, pilloried by society and told that AIDS was their own fault, were utterly non-judgmental themselves. It's a lesson I've tried to adopt in my own life ever since.

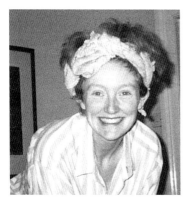

"We had the whole cast of *East Enders* pulling pints in the pubs, Boy George in the Rock Garden, Jonathan Ross in Paul Smith's clothes shop, Kate Bush was there, Harry Enfield…"

When any of them died, it was devastating for the group. I went to fifteen funerals in the space of nine months. Many of them had been shunned by their own families, thrown out onto the street, so they were making their own family among themselves, as gay men do.

I wanted to use my theatre connections to raise money for them so, that winter, 1987, I and some theatre friends went round all the stage doors and organised a charity gala called *Thingathon* where the West End shows came together on a Sunday for a whole day, singing and dancing. Everyone was happy to give their time and do their ten-minute slot. It sold out very quickly.

But I thought we could go further to try and reach the kind of people who wouldn't go to theatres. I came up with the idea of enlisting a load of celebrities to take over the Piazza at Covent Garden, with all its shops and restaurants and pubs, for a day. We called it *Shop Assistance* and it took nearly a year to organise. When I first approached the shops and pubs in Covent Garden, the majority gave me a flat *No*. No way did they want to be associated with this "gay plague", as one put it: we were dealing

with a huge amount of fear and homophobia. But I was itching for a battle. I wanted to make a difference and I wasn't going to take no for an answer. I made them all hear my story about myself and Geoffrey, how I'd given up my career to do this and that it was everybody's responsibility to help us.

I had a wonderful team of friends helping me, a remarkable bunch who have gone on effectively to run British theatre between them. J. Walter Thompson, the big ad agency, designed and printed a poster for free. We had the whole cast of *East Enders* pulling pints in the pubs, Boy George in the Rock Garden, Jonathan Ross in Paul Smith's clothes shop, Kate Bush was there, Harry Enfield did his *LoadsaMoney* comedy routine… we ended up with about 250 celebrities helping that day across the whole Covent Garden area. Boy George was wonderful. People wanted his autograph, but he refused to sign unless they donated money, and he made sure each of them went away with an information leaflet about HIV.

That same year, 1988, I instigated bucket collections in all the West End theatres on World Aids Day, 1st December. After the curtain call, whoever was the show's star would bring one of the Frontliners group on stage, introduce them and they would tell their story. They were nervous, of course, but the cast always treated them like royalty.

I spent most of that year, it seemed, counting coins and cash. Once I and a volunteer were driving to the Barbican with a car loaded with heavy buckets of coins, and a policeman stopped us. He made us open the boot, took one look and the eyebrow went up. We explained who were and what the money was. I don't think he could decide whether to believe us or not, so he insisted on coming to the Barbican with us to check we hadn't nicked it!

After two years, I suppose I'd burnt myself out and lost the energy and spark that had fuelled me. One of the Frontliners saw how drained I was and sat me down with a cup of coffee. "Kelly," he said, "I saw you as Sally Bowles in *Cabaret*. You have a talent most of us would give our left arms for. Don't you think it's time to go back to doing what you do so brilliantly, singing and dancing and acting?"

I assured him my place was there, raising money, but couldn't stop thinking about what he'd said. Two months later when he died, I started to feel it was time to go back to my career.

"I wonder if we'd be able to do today what we did then. We see so many horrors every day in the news that too many of us have compassion fatigue. People have lost sight of the bigger picture…"

I wonder if we'd be able to do today what we did then. We see so many horrors every day in the news that too many of us have compassion fatigue. People have lost sight of the bigger picture – they obsess about themselves and their rights, instead of thinking about their responsibilities as individuals to help others. Everything happens through the filter of social media and if someone gets involved with a cause, they immediately get trolled as 'interfering do-gooders'.

But those life lessons I absorbed as a young woman of 23, working with those wonderful men, have stayed with me ever since and inform how I live my life.

"I think of them all now, and remember what we achieved together."

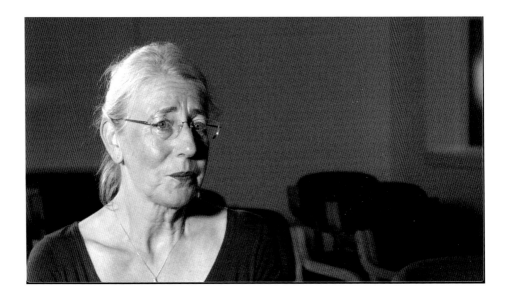

"Patients with HIV deserved to be treated as human beings, but instead they were met with prejudice and fear."

Jane Bruton began her nursing career in Leicester and first encountered HIV patients when she became Ward Sister in the infectious diseases unit there. After a short spell as a health advisor in the Sexual Health Clinic at the Chelsea and Westminster Hospital, in 1989 she became Sister on Broderip Ward, the dedicated HIV ward at the Middlesex Hospital. Jane returned to the Chelsea and Westminster in 1999 for a further 14 years in various Senior Nurse roles in HIV. She has also worked with HIV patients in rural Uganda, and she is now the Clinical Research Manager in the Patient Experience Research Centre at Imperial College, London.

"Close contact was what these young men needed … it was reassuring to be looked after by someone familiar who became a friend."

AIDS revolutionised the way patients were cared for in hospital, and some of the changes persist to this day.

Jane Bruton
"When there's no cure, all you can do is care."

My career began just as a quiet revolution in nursing care was getting underway in the NHS. Old-style nursing was task-orientated, bringing bedpans, changing sheets, but the new approach was based on looking after the person as a whole. It offered a huge opportunity to make a difference to the lives of patients with HIV, whom I felt had been poorly treated. The Ward Sister I took over from in the Infectious Diseases Unit was an old-school martinet – strict about visiting, not at all empathetic. I was determined to make a change. The first patient I nursed with HIV there was terribly isolated, frightened and sad, in his despair refusing to talk to anyone. He had a disfiguring fungal infection in his nails and no-one had made any effort to get close to him or give him an opportunity to open up. I went into his room and just sat with him, until eventually he began to talk.

Patients with HIV deserved to be treated as human beings, but instead they were met with prejudice and fear. One had been working in the shoe industry, and thought he should act responsibly and let his employers know that he was HIV positive, in case he ever cut himself on the machines. The next day, he'd lost his job. I had endless confrontations with ambulance staff. The drivers who brought patients to our ward had been ferrying infectious patients there for years without a qualm. But as soon as they had to transport an HIV patient, they would insist on wearing full protective gear, dressed like spacemen for fear of contamination. Some of my nursing staff threatened to walk out when I arranged for them to have gay awareness sessions with the Leicester AIDS Support Society, but the sessions did make a difference to how they nursed the patients.

Leicester had only a few patients with HIV, but my next job brought me into contact with people living with HIV every day, as a Health Advisor in the sexual health clinic at Chelsea and Westminster. My role was to support people through the process of being tested for HIV. It was important to discuss, before they tested, whether they were ready to receive an HIV diagnosis, which was at

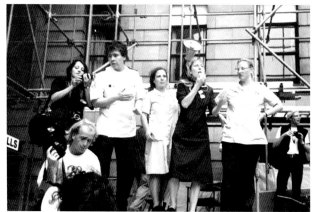

"Even if I'd wanted to, I doubt I could have stopped the kissing and hugging."

Jane (holding megaphone) & colleagues on a picket line

that time effectively a death sentence. One young woman fainted when I gave her the diagnosis. Some didn't feel ready to go through with the test and, if they didn't come back, we wouldn't chase them. If they were diagnosed as HIV positive, we would refer them to the Kobler Clinic next door and continue to offer them support. We might even go with them when they broke the news to a partner or to family. All this gave me invaluable insights for working with AIDS patients in my next post.

Broderip Ward at the Middlesex had been opened by Princess Diana in 1987, two years before I became Ward Sister there. The plaque on the wall that commemorated the opening was kept covered by a painting, to conceal this was an HIV ward, because some wanted to keep the nature of their illness secret. There were four single rooms, plus eight beds in the main Nightingale-style ward. It was full of people with pneumocystis pneumonia, lymphoma, cryptococcal meningitis, toxoplasmosis or any of the multiple opportunistic infections that AIDS patients might develop. But it was like no other ward I'd ever worked on. The first thing the consultants said to me when I arrived was: "Jane, the nurses kiss and hug the patients all the time – could you do something about it?"

Even if I'd wanted to, I doubt I could have stopped the kissing and hugging. Close contact was what these young men needed, ostracised by so many outside who were afraid to touch them. The nursing staff were either young women, like myself, without children, or gay men, and naturally we felt empathy. There was a kind of siege mentality – us against the world – especially when hate mail arrived or the press tried to sneak in, disguised as visitors. After a patient was discharged, our nurses would often have to look after them at home too, finishing the day shift then taking groceries round or changing their dressings, because the district nurses wouldn't help an AIDS patient. No wonder we grew close.

66

On the other hand, boundaries did need to be looked at, to ensure staff didn't burn out. It was easy to become too involved, and this was the toughest kind of nursing there is. When a new patient came onto the ward, you knew that within a few months or a year, you could be holding their hand as they died, although they were no older than yourself.

"When a new patient came onto the ward, you knew that within a few months or a year, you could be holding their hand as they died…"

When there's no cure, all you can do is care. We nursed in teams. Each team had its own group of patients to look after, and each nurse within the team would be given special responsibility for their patient from admission to discharge, and for any subsequent returns to the ward. Our patients were often anxious and fearful, and the continuity was soothing. They wouldn't have to keep repeating their story to a new set of nurses every time. Some of the procedures we put them through were invasive and gruelling: bronchoscopy, lumbar puncture and the like. They might feel humiliated by the way AIDS took over their body, with uncontrollable diarrhoea, or the swelling and disfigurement of Kaposi's sarcoma; it was reassuring to be looked after by someone familiar who became a friend.

"What was special on Broderip was the levelling of relationships between patients, nurses and doctors."

What was special on Broderip was the levelling of relationships between patients, nurses and doctors. The hierarchy was flattened to the extent that it might be hard to tell, when you arrived on the ward, who was who. We dispensed with uniforms. We always used to wear our own clothes at Christmas, so I thought, why don't we do it all the time? We consulted the patients – a few wanted us in proper nurses' uniforms with hat and frills and apron, but most were delighted to see us in mufti. It sparked no end of conversations about who was wearing what today, or what colour the staff nurse had dyed his hair and beard – once, green. Even the domestic cleaner on our ward was very much a part of the team. Jacinta would always be there if we had a party or a night out with patients.

Apart from medical treatment, our job was to enable people to live their lives as fully as possible. I made sure we had decent china cups and plates for the patients to eat off, a fridge full of treats, subtle illumination from bedside lamps

"Apart from medical treatment, our job was to enable people to live their lives as fully as possible."

rather than the harsh glare of overhead lighting. There were a lot of parties and, if a patient couldn't get out of bed, we'd wheel them over to join in. At Christmas, the nurses would cook Christmas dinner themselves and share it with the patients. It had to be special because, for many, it would be their last Christmas dinner.

One man was a singer and a dancer in musical theatre. He'd been admitted with cryptococcal meningitis and had been very sick. His temperature was still sky-high on the day his agent rang about an audition for a show he'd always wanted to perform in. He was desperate to audition, but we knew the consultant would almost certainly refuse to let him go in the state he was in. We dosed him up with paracetamol to get his temperature down, and when it came to the ward round, we steered the consultant smartly past the bed, as I said brightly: "Look how far his temperature has dropped!" So off he went to the audition and he got the part. It seemed to give him a new lease of life. The rest of the cast knew about his diagnosis and supported him through the production, and a bed was made up in the dressing room so he could rest between scenes. Towards the end of the show's run, he became weaker and wasn't up to all the singing and dancing, but they gave him a smaller part so he could continue appearing on stage. I went to his funeral, in the Actors' Church in Covent Garden, where the cast sang numbers from the show. It was the most wonderful send off for this talented man.

"We wanted to give people the best death possible."

We wanted to give people the best death possible. Living wills, or patient directives, as they're often known, came about because HIV patients wanted some control over their treatment as they became more ill. They enabled us to discuss how we should care for them if they became comatosed or their heart stopped – would they want to be revived or not? Who should we call? These frank conversations about end of life helped them cope with their fears around dying and, of course, they were very afraid, something that got to me more than anything else. I remember one patient who had always been very dapper, in beautiful Italian suits, who picked out the clothes he wanted to be dressed in after he died. Sadly, he'd lost a lot of weight, so the suit was huge on him. The mismatch between who he had been, and what he had become when he died, broke my heart.

"We learned to listen to patients… to give them space to talk about their fears. Above all, we learned to see them as individuals, as people."

We learned to listen to patients and to provide what they needed. We learned to give them space to talk about their fears. Above all, we learned to see them as individuals, as people. What we learned from caring for those young men was a way of nursing that can't always be replicated under today's pressures in the NHS, but which has left a very real legacy in hospitals today.

1981 marked the beginning of a pandemic that has seen 76 million infected with the HIV virus and 33 million die (WHO statistics). The COVID-19 pandemic is on a different scale and speed from HIV in the 1980s and 1990s, but while there are many differences, there are similarities too and lessons from HIV that can usefully be shared. During the first wave I read a post on a social media site from a nurse working with COVID-19 patients: she describes how the care team "had never felt so close and supportive" from the consultant to the cleaner. She described nurses working extra hours to support each other despite their worries. Finally, she talked about how, with scared patients and no family allowed, nurses had to be "more than healthcare workers" for the patient and the family. It felt like I was reading about my ward 30 years ago.

There is, or rather should be, no going back once you have experienced a levelling of the team, valuing each and every role and person on the team, and developing those deeper relationships with patients and family. I say 'should be' because we lost some of those gains in the nursing model when new antiretroviral treatments presaged a more medical model approach. Despite this, nurses have continued to develop and promote patient-centred care and value team working.

It must be hard now for nurses on the front line of COVID-19 work to reflect on what's happening. All they can do is get through each day, working extra hours, supporting each other, getting exhausted and yet not able to sleep.

Right now, no-one knows when the right time will be to begin reflection. But from my experience in acute HIV, the wounds being inflicted today will run deep. For us, formal reflection, through recording oral histories from nurses and other healthcare workers, has been very important.

"That is the value of telling our stories now."

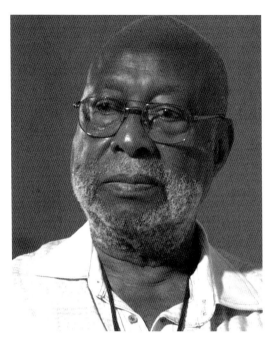

"Were there people in the black community suffering from this illness? ... I decided to try to find them and set up some sort of support they would use."

Arnold Gordon was born in Sierra Leone and began a broadcasting career in the UK with the BBC's African Service, before returning to Sierra Leone in the 1980s to run the television service there. He was contacted by a friend in the UK who had contracted HIV/AIDS, which prompted him to return to London and volunteer with the Terrence Higgins Trust. He went on to found Blackliners, an HIV support group for the black community, and eventually went on to work as a marriage guidance counsellor, before retiring to Kent where he writes about the legacy of slavery and how it affected his own family in Sierra Leone.

"But there was a huge appetite among young, gay, black men for what we could do to help them. They wanted counselling and they needed condoms ..."

Blackliners grew out of a realisation that there were no organisations dealing with HIV that catered specifically for the black community, with the result that many HIV+ black people in the UK felt side-lined. Arnold describes the role the charity played in raising awareness and supporting the black community in various ways.

Arnold Gordon

"… there was a great deal of stigma attached to HIV in the black community."

My friend, who eventually died from AIDS, pointed out to me that I had been lucky to escape HIV simply by virtue of being out of the country while the pandemic struck, because our lifestyles had been very similar. He persuaded me to volunteer as a buddy with the Terrence Higgins Trust. I used to visit a young man who lived alone in a high rise flat in Docklands, whose friends had deserted him. I would take him to the pub once a week to have a drink and a chat, though he needed to be coaxed because his face was disfigured with Kaposi's Sarcoma and he was shy about being seen. He would sit in the corner with his cap pulled down. When he died, I went to his funeral, and all his old mates turned up, claiming they hadn't realised how ill he was. I felt like punching them in the face.

THT was doing an impressive job, but it struck me that everyone who came through the door was white, male and gay. Were there people in the black community suffering from this illness? We didn't see any of them, but I knew there had to be, so I decided to try to find them and set up some sort of support they would use.

Blackliners began in 1988 as a telephone helpline set up in the spare room in my flat in Balham. Once the word went out, calls built up and before long we had to find funding for an office in Brixton and set ourselves up as a charity. We soon realised there was a great deal of stigma attached to HIV in the black community. I once managed to persuade Doctor John Sentamu, who later went on to become Archbishop of York but was then in charge of a church in Herne Hill, to preach a sermon on compassion for National AIDS Day. Afterwards older members of his congregation made it plain that they didn't want to hear about such things.

But there was a huge appetite among young, gay, black men for what we could do to help them. They wanted counselling and they needed condoms, because few were using them at that point. One man I talked to told me he had one

> **"From counselling and condoms, we went on to help with housing."**

> **"… we were also dealing with the breakdown of relationships, both gay and straight, when a partner discovered the other had HIV …"**

condom which he would wash and wear, over and over again, because he couldn't afford to buy more! We gave them out for free at the office.

From counselling and condoms, we went on to help with housing. One Christmas Eve, we were closing the office when a distressed young boy came in to tell us he'd been thrown out of the house because his parents had found out he was gay and HIV positive. He had nowhere to go, so one of our volunteers took him in over Christmas. It highlighted that we needed somewhere to accommodate people like him. We contacted a local Housing Association and looked for funding from one of the big construction companies. They told us: "Find the land and we'll build something." We secured a plot in Wandsworth where they built us six one-roomed bungalows and equipped them.

By this time, we were also dealing with the breakdown of relationships, both gay and straight, when a partner discovered the other had HIV. Heterosexual couples turned to us: perhaps a wife who discovered her husband was sleeping around and wanted advice on how to stay safe from HIV, or how to be tested. The saddest case was a man from Uganda who passed the virus on to his wife, but was in denial so he accused *her* of sleeping around. He beat her up, she died and he went to prison. The prison contacted us, and one of our counsellors went in once a week to talk to him, and to bring him familiar African food to replace what the prison service could offer. Food for black people in hospital became another project. An African restaurant in Brixton would make up a week's worth of meal cartons which were taken to hospitals to be kept in their freezers and served as needed. Deaths were frequent. At this time, there were no drugs to combat the virus apart from AZT, and not everyone was able to tolerate it. I stopped going to funerals after a while – it was too harrowing.

The work was stressful, especially as time went on and it seemed that people were becoming complacent about the risks. I remember younger black guys saying:

"Nothing to do with us, it's those who went to America and brought it back to the UK – they're all dead and gone now, so why should we worry?" Or – and this was a line I particularly hated – "Nothing to do with us, it's a white man's disease." The wider black community was hostile to our work because they felt we were stigmatising black people – remember, this was a time when all sorts of ridiculous and offensive myths were circulating about how AIDS had transferred into humans through Africans having sex with monkeys.

At the height of our success, we were dealing with people as far afield as Manchester, opening an outreach office there, and one in Bristol where there is a large and diverse black community. Mel C from the Spice Girls threw a huge party in her house for us, and raised around a hundred thousand pounds from her friends.

I eventually retired and left Blackliners in the hands of others, but though it has now been subsumed into the wider work of the Terrence Higgins Trust, I'm immensely proud of the organisation I founded, which made such a difference to the lives of black people living with HIV and AIDS. It's a contribution I am grateful to have been able to make to my community.

> "The wider black community was hostile to our work because they felt we were stigmatising black people."

> "I'm immensely proud of the organisation I founded, which made such a difference to the lives of black people living with HIV and AIDS."

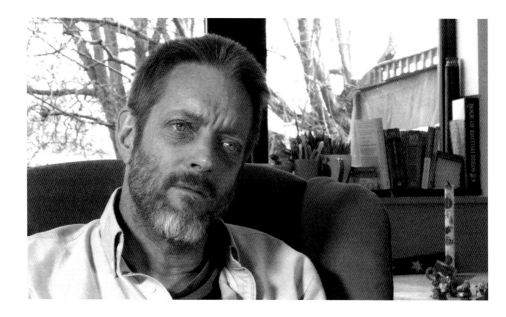

"That's when it hits you that this is not some ghetto condition affecting just one group of people; this is everybody. We are all in this."

Richard Leaf is an English writer who went to university in San Francisco and lived there from 1978 to 1983, working after he graduated in theatre. He returned to the UK in 1983 to go to drama school and then joined the Royal Shakespeare Company. He has appeared in films such as *Braveheart, Hannibal Rising, The Fifth Element, Harry Potter and The Order of The Phoenix.*

"… our value is our humanity, shared with other people…"

Richard Leaf witnessed the earliest days of the AIDS pandemic in San Francisco in the early 1980s as an outsider, a straight man. In the 1990s, he began volunteering at the Mildmay Hospice and the memory of the people he encountered there will remain with him for ever.

Richard Leaf
"Unconditional love …"

S an Francisco at the end of the 1970s and into the 1980s was the most wonderful, freeing place to be. It was a revelation: joyous, confrontational, liberal, terrific fun. My girlfriend at the time hung out on the fringes of the gay scene and took me to Polk and Castro. You would go down to Castro on Hallowe'en, and I'd never seen anything like it. It was incredible street-theatre. I remember one guy dressed as a PanAm stewardess, waltzing down the street, "Please fasten your seatbelts", doing the whole routine, or The Sisters of Perpetual Indulgence, a group of gay men dressed as nuns who raised money for charity.

I was completely naïve about gay sexuality at the time, being straight and essentially monogamous. I had a job for a while painting the front of a toyshop owned by two gay guys who were a couple. They gave me *carte blanche* to make it as colourful as I could – gold and green, yellow and blue and purple. Every lunchtime, one would leave the shop and go up to the park for lunch. Then he'd come back, and the other would leave and go to the park. I thought it curious, and it was only when my girlfriend explained it to me that I understood. That was San Francisco – a tangible atmosphere of anything goes.

But there were also pockets of redneck prejudice in the city, people with long hair and beards who would spit in your face if they thought you

> "It was a revelation: joyous, confrontational, liberal, terrific fun. … It was incredible street-theatre."

> "I would be called 'faggot' and have stones thrown at me."

"Then one day, people you worked with in the theatre there suddenly stopped coming into work."

looked different. I had short hair and an earring, and wore suits with skinny ties, and I would be called 'faggot' and have stones thrown at me. Not long after I arrived in the city, Harvey Milk, a local politician and gay activist, was assassinated along with the Mayor, George Moscone, who'd signed a bill outlawing discrimination against gays.

Then one day, people you worked with in the theatre there suddenly stopped coming into work. They would disappear into a black hole. We didn't know what was wrong with them. People died very quickly, and horror stories began to circulate, about the lesions, emaciation, people's skin falling off.

I remember sitting in a friend's house, having my hair cut. A TV evangelist appeared on the screen and said: "AIDS is God's vengeance on the gay community." It made me feel sick. The men dying might have had the kind of lifestyle I didn't, but they didn't deserve this.

After my visa and my money ran out and I went home, letters from friends in San Francisco kept arriving, telling of more illness among people we knew, more deaths.

"… to come to a place like that day-centre where they could be open and recognised for who they were, was a release."

There was a palpable sense of fear too among the gay people I worked with in UK theatre. We were all shocked when, in 1990, the actor Ian Charleson died. I was between acting jobs and my first marriage had broken down, so I started doing voluntary work almost as a kind of therapy really, to take my mind off my own problems. After a stint at a homeless hostel, I became involved with the Mildmay Hospice in Shoreditch, where a friend of mine had a job.

The Mildmay had a day-care centre where I spent most of my time, but they also had in-patient rooms for respite care, or when people were reaching the end. I'd make cups of tea, give people their lunch, fetch their medication from the pharmacy and hear their stories.

At that time, having AIDS and HIV was a terrible stigma. People tried to hide that they had it, because rumours circulated among the public about how it could be caught from tears or sweat, which was rubbish. For our clients, to come to a place like that day-centre where they could be open and recognised for who they were, was a release. I was a churchgoer and Mildmay was a Christian organisation. But the real embodiment of Christ, that unconditional love that transcends everything, was in those people who came to the day centre. They were staring at a death sentence because there was no cure. It was only a matter of time and they all knew it: they had the lesions, they grew thin, then they were gone. But their generosity towards each other was without parallel in my experience.

AIDS has its peaks and troughs and, whenever someone hit a trough, the friends they'd made at the Mildmay would do whatever they could to help them through. They were indefatigable in the service of each other. They would walk across town to encourage and support each other, cooking their food, sitting holding their hands. They were all on benefits because they could no longer work so, to save money, they would walk everywhere instead of taking the bus or tube, and it took its toll on their feet. I admired them for their bluntness. They would come in and say, I'm having a shit day, can someone please come and bathe my feet? It was a privilege to do it.

As well as gay men there were also women, drug users or Africans or simply people whose partners had passed the virus to them. That's when it hits you that this is not some ghetto condition affecting just one group of people; this is everybody. We are all in this.

One of my jobs was to go round the wards and ask people if they'd like a priest to give them Holy Communion. I remember knocking on one door to see an African gentleman in his pyjamas, shaving his cheek to try to maintain some sort of dignity, some

"They were staring at a death sentence because there was no cure. … But their generosity towards each other was without parallel in my experience."

> "I'd never witnessed someone so caught between their struggle to be seen as human, and their fear of what was happening to them."

> "Those examples of unconditional love at the Mildmay have stayed with me forever. I've forgotten almost all of their names, because I'm hopeless at names, but those faces, they never leave me."

fading sense of the person he'd been before his illness.

He turned and looked at me with his face full of awful shame because of the way he looked. His whole lip was peeling off, like someone sloughing their skin, a horrific sight. He told me yes, he would like Communion, but I'd never witnessed someone so caught between their struggle to be seen as human, and their fear of what was happening to them.

Another time, I knocked on a door and went in to find pitch darkness, like a pit. You could sense the rage in the room. When I asked if the person there would like to take Communion, a howl of raw anger came from the bed: "Aaarghhh f——— ooooooff…." Furious, terrified. That sort of moment never leaves you.

Many, many people have done much, much more than I did, more tirelessly, more selflessly, trying to find a cure so people can have hope and get better. But what I took from my experience at the Mildmay is that our value isn't dependent on our bank account or our status in society or the job we do; our value is our humanity, shared with other people. In the face of equally insurmountable troubles, especially these days when times are strange and turning, the thing we can all do is the thing right in front of us, to hold out our hand to the next person who needs help. If you're blinded by the tsunami of horror coming at you, you will be nothing more than driftwood.

Those examples of unconditional love at the Mildmay have stayed with me forever. I've forgotten almost all of their names, because I'm hopeless at names, but those faces, they never leave me.

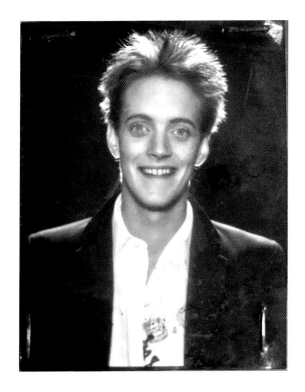

"… the thing we can all do is the thing right in front of us, to hold out our hand to the next person who needs help. If you're blinded by the tsunami of horror coming at you, you will be nothing more than driftwood."

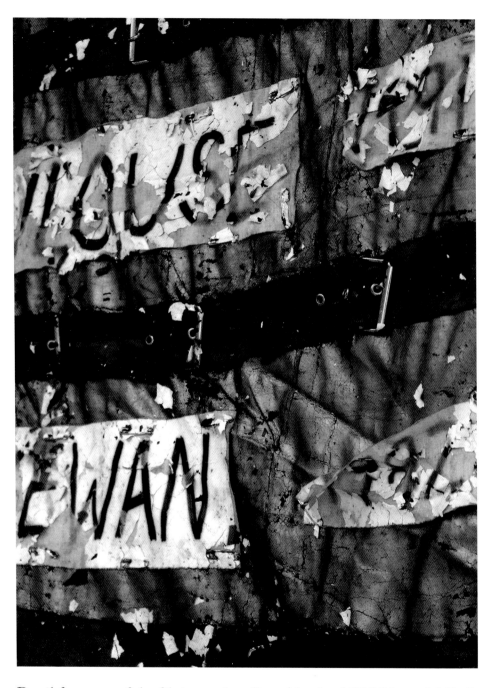

Detail from one of the fabric panels collected by the AIDS Memorial Quilt Preservation Partnership.

Part II: 1991–1999
"Pressures on the levers of scientific power…"

Ryan White, aged 18 – who had been banned from school in the US – died in 1990 from AIDS-related complications. In 1991, the year the red ribbon became a symbol to signify awareness and support for people living with HIV/AIDS, Freddie Mercury announced that he was living with AIDS and died the following day. In the US, the basketball player Magic Johnson announced his retirement after being diagnosed with HIV. His subsequent campaigns on the subject helped dispel the widely held belief that the risk of HIV infection was limited to the gay community. Similarly, tennis star Arthur Ashe's announcement of his diagnosis through a blood transfusion in 1992 served to challenge stigma and demystify the condition. Although AZT had been approved for use as an antiretroviral drug in 1987, there was still no effective medical treatment for the virus. But change was on the horizon.

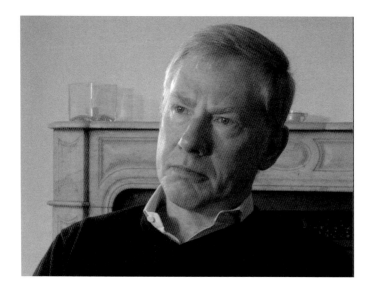

"... a positive HIV test was also the thief of hopes and dreams ..."

Dr Graeme Moyle graduated from medical school in Adelaide, Australia in 1986. His interest in infectious diseases led him in 1988 to the UK to specialise in HIV medicine and research. Much of his career has been associated with the Kobler Clinic in London, part of Chelsea and Westminster Hospital, but he also spent two years working in the pharmaceutical industry helping develop one of a new generation of HIV drugs. He is now Director of HIV Research at the Chelsea and Westminster Hospital.

"The social workers ... to help patients claim disability benefits now found themselves helping many return to work."

In the 1980s, when Graeme Moyle began work in HIV clinics, a diagnosis of HIV typically shortened life expectancy by 40 years. Through the commitment of the pharmaceutical industry and some Governmental bodies, such as the US National Institutes of Health, and the willingness of people with HIV to participate in clinical trials, treatments and diagnostic tools progressively improved until, in 1996, new classes of medications, the protease inhibitors and non-nucleoside reverse transcriptase inhibitors, along with enhanced abilities to test for viral load, were able to turn the tide. Combinations of medications were found to suppress the virus leading to dramatic changes in individuals' health, quality of life and life expectancy. This essay looks at the progress in treatment and drug development from the clinician's viewpoint.

Dr Graeme Moyle
"HIV brought about a reinvention in medicine …"

In the mid-1990s, two critical developments changed everything for people with HIV. The first was the ability to directly measure viral activity or viral load. The second was combination therapy that included new drugs with novel mechanisms of action and which had a profound impact on viral load. To our relief, we at last began to see patients beginning to get better, instead of spiralling inevitably downwards.

This was very different from when I started to work in HIV medicine. In 1988, things were very grim indeed. Although a few HIV patients get sick quite rapidly, the average time from acquiring the virus to becoming ill was, typically, eight to ten years. Most people went through a period where they were relatively or completely well and unaware they'd been infected, but still able to pass on the virus to others. People were often reticent about testing, because it simply revealed they were infected with something untreatable and unmasked the likelihood of soon becoming ill and dying early; a positive HIV test was also the thief of hopes and dreams. The CDC definition of HIV disease led only one way: well to ill, to AIDS, to death.

"We, as doctors, were dealing with something much more overwhelming, in terms of numbers of infections and severity of their immune deficiency, than we had ever dealt with before …"

People would often present with something mild but persistent – thrush in their mouth, white marks on the side of their tongue, skin problems. Others would present with the hallmarks of AIDS, such as unusual pneumonias, a viral infection in the eye, or the disfiguring Kaposi's sarcoma on their face. All we could do to help was to treat those infections, with antibiotics, antivirals or other standard medication. With each new infection, they would accumulate more and more treatments, more tablets, more injections, more intravenous infusions, with all the concomitant side effects: rashes, nausea, diarrhoea, anaemia, weight loss. We, as doctors, were dealing with something much more overwhelming, in terms of numbers of infections and severity of their immune deficiency, than we had ever dealt with before or seen described in medical literature. We had a thousand patients on our books for whom we might need 30, 40 or 50 beds at any one time, and we could expect to see five patients a week dying. But we were diagnosing as many as ten new patients a week, so numbers were growing. This was just one clinic of several in London, many more across the country.

The Kobler, part funded by a generous donation, was a purpose-built block separate from the main St Stephen's Hospital, subsequently rebuilt as the Chelsea and Westminster Hospital. It was close to Earl's Court, whose pubs and clubs were one of the centres for gay life in London, but even in the early days we also saw many women, as well as people from some more established risk groups such as people from high prevalence countries in sub-Saharan Africa, people who had injected drugs, as well as people who had no clear idea how they may have acquired HIV. Often the only risk factor for acquiring HIV is that they have been sexually active, and we know the majority of HIV transmission globally is heterosexual.

"Often the only risk factor for acquiring HIV is that they have been sexually active, and we know the majority of HIV transmission globally is heterosexual."

We made sure the physical environment was sympathetic to patients' needs – soft, comfortable chairs, for instance, for wasted, bony posteriors. None of the doctors wore gowns or white coats. Our philosophy was to wear street clothes to break down the doctor–patient barrier. Volunteers provided tea, coffee and cakes. We had our own onsite pharmacy so people who had difficulty walking didn't have far to go to pick up medication, and our own day care unit for infusions and onsite diagnostic facilities, so endoscopies and other tests could be performed there instead of having to make arrangements in the main hospital.

An equally important part of our work was recognising there is a balance between length of life and quality of life … and ensuring someone's quality of death was good when that time came. What's the point in continuing on toxic medication if you only have weeks to live? I remember one patient who went out to buy the best pair of silk pyjamas he could find, a luxury he'd not enjoyed before, so he could die in them. People faced their premature death with such dignity and nobility, often supported by friends and loved ones who knew their time was also running low.

By the early 1990s, many of the bars and clubs in Earl's Court were closing and the London Apprentice pub in Old Street had already shut because, effectively, its entire clientele was dead. It is estimated that 70% of the gay men from the Earl's Court area died, a bigger impact on a community than, for instance, a village whose young men went off to fight in the First World War. A whole generation of gay men was wiped out by HIV, beautiful, creative, talented, loved young men. Think what they might have achieved with the 40 years of life stolen from them. Society is the poorer for their passing.

That more *didn't* die is largely down to the efforts of the gay community themselves, who were active in promoting messages around safe sex and placing pressure on the levers of scientific power, so the development of new treatments became a priority. As a result, we now have a gay community in London which is mostly HIV free, and we limited an expansion of HIV more broadly into the UK's population.

The only treatment for the virus when I started in 1988 was AZT, an important development because it proved that a weak antiviral drug could buy time. Unfortunately, it didn't extend life by much, because the virus became resistant to it and, as we gave it in high doses, hoping for greater effect, it often made people sicker than before. But it became an important building block for adding new antivirals as they were invented. My job was a mixture of clinical care and research, because we wanted to get new drugs out to patients as fast as they became available. The way to do that is through clinical trials, before drugs are licensed or approved. Through that process, HIV brought about a reinvention in medicine. Because so many were dying, we had to put our foot on the accelerator very rapidly. Something very similar has

"A whole generation of gay men was wiped out by HIV, beautiful, creative, talented, loved young men. Think what they might have achieved with the 40 years of life stolen from them. Society is the poorer for their passing."

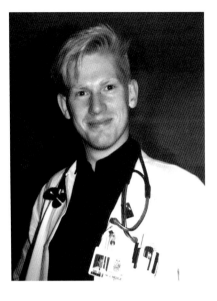

been happening during the coronavirus pandemic, where patients willingly consent to what are still experimental treatments.

At the Kobler, we did some of the first studies looking at combination therapy and were involved in the development of viral load testing. When we began combining drugs, going from one to two, we saw a small improvement in people's CD4 numbers – that is, the T-cells that help fight infection. Unfortunately, there was also an increase in the amount of side effects so, as we began trials using three drugs instead of two, we were not expecting any significant improvement. How wrong we were.

The watershed moment was July 1996, at the World AIDS Conference in Vancouver. Several groups reported on clinical studies where, starting on three drugs at the same time, patients' viral load dropped below the limits of what could be measured – and remained there. Alongside came remarkable improvement in their CD4 cell counts. From the moment we began using triple therapy routinely in the UK, we saw what we called the 'Lazarus' phenomenon. People we'd thought would die had their health restored. The social workers employed at the Kobler to help patients claim disability benefits now found themselves helping many return to work. A patient of mine, whom I'd advised to take early retirement and make his will, started on triple therapy involving a protease inhibitor called Indinavir, and described starting his new 'cocktail' as if someone was turning off the switches on his switchboard of symptoms. One by one, they went away – the night sweats, the fatigue, the weight loss, the diarrhoea, until two years later he was able to return to his profession and rise to the very top of it.

Now, 25 years later, side effects from the medication have been vastly diminished as we have refined treatments and expended options. People are less fearful of diagnosis and stigma, while still a problem, has diminished. We are at a point where, provided we diagnose HIV early enough, we can rapidly reduce viral load to undetectable levels and safely say that person can no longer transmit HIV: "undetectable = untransmissible."Additional, PrEP – pre-exposure prophylaxis – is available for people whose activity puts them at risk of the virus.

But to suggest HIV is no longer a problem would be naïve. Donations, that funded much of the care and were at their peak when many people were dying through HIV, are drying up. Studies of how people age with HIV already reveal that those who've been infected the longest and exposed to the older generation of treatments, tend to carry a bigger burden of health issues into old age than the general population – a greater chance of high blood pressure, diabetes, kidney disease, heart attacks, cognitive disturbances. The precise cause is not yet clear: some of it may relate to the virus, some to medications they received in the past as well as lifestyle factors such as smoking, alcohol and recreational substances.

Above and beyond, there is also the question of how surviving HIV has affected mental health. In the early 1980s, a gay man called Stephen Crohn was the partner of one of the first people to die in New York of AIDS. Crohn had been exposed many times to the virus, through his partners, yet he never became infected and seemed to be uninfectable. It turned out he had a genetic variation in his CD4 cells, missing a receptor called CCR5 for the virus to latch onto. Over the years, he assisted scientists, who were eventually able to use his genetic variation to develop a new treatment and, via a bone marrow transplant in one individual, an apparent 'cure' for HIV. But in 2013, aged 66, Crohn committed suicide. The note he left explained the burden of being the last one of his friends left, of having photo albums and diaries recording the fabulous lives of people who had died long ago in the glow of their youth. He had lost his social network, those people with whom he would otherwise have grown old disgracefully, and he couldn't live with that knowledge.

"Sadly, for a generation of people now reaching their 60s and 70s, growing old without a wide and strong social and support network is the next challenge in the long list of things HIV has thrown at them."

"As a result, we now have a gay community in London which is mostly HIV free, and we limited an expansion of HIV more broadly into the UK's population."

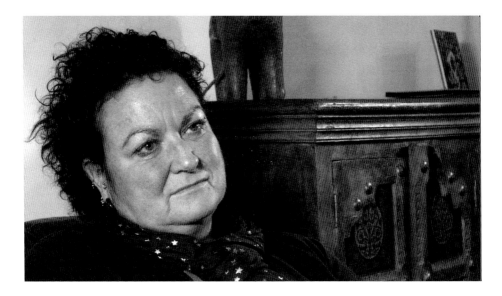

"We were ... writing the book as we went along, but it was about treating people with respect and dignity, seeing the person as the primary point of care."

Flick Thorley was born in New Zealand, and trained there as a nurse in the mid-1980s. She came to the UK in 1989, and began working as a psychiatric nurse at University College Hospital (UCH) in London. She became a charge nurse at the London Lighthouse, and later worked on the HIV ward at the Chelsea and Westminster Hospital, where she was also instrumental in setting up a club drugs clinic. She and her partner, Chloe Orkin, a consultant also working in the field of HIV and AIDS, were seconded to Botswana to set up an antiretroviral programme there for HIV sufferers. Flick has retired from the NHS but now volunteers with her dogs, offering pet therapy in hospices.

In the early years of the AIDS pandemic, the focus was on the physical needs of people with the illness. But by the 1990s it was becoming clear that people with AIDS could also become acutely psychiatrically unwell, often as a result of the illness attacking the brain, and that the NHS didn't have the facilities to cope with this aspect of the condition. Flick Thorley recalls the pioneering work she was involved with at that time which helped remedy the situation, and the care given by the London Lighthouse.

Flick Thorley

"Some lived so long in the expectation they'd die, they couldn't cope with surviving …"

As a psychiatric nurse, the first person I looked after who was HIV positive was a young boy with psychosis in a psychiatric hospital in New Zealand and it was, to put it mildly, a disaster. We were scared of it and scared of him. I feel ashamed, looking back, of how we treated him, because he was just a frightened, ill kid whom we kept in an isolation room, and barrier-nursed, double-gloved, double-gowned. His cutlery was plastic, he ate off paper plates, and we burned his bedding. Even then, I realised that the way he was treated was unacceptable, but at the time we just didn't know how to handle this terrifying illness.

By the early 1990s I was a nurse on one of the acute psychiatric wards at UCH in London. A young gay man with advanced HIV was transferred to us, because the HIV ward at the Middlesex could no longer cope with him. He was psychotic and demented, with brain lesions caused by HIV, and he was dying. We couldn't cope either, because we weren't set up to deal with the physical side of his illness, such as uncontrollable diarrhoea. Here I was again, trying to nurse someone in a completely inappropriate setting for their condition, because there was no appropriate place. He couldn't be at home safely, he couldn't be on a medical ward safely, he couldn't be in a psychiatric hospital safely, and he didn't know where he was but he knew he didn't want to be there.

The upshot was that he was moved back to the Middlesex and I became a liaison nurse between the HIV ward there and the psychiatric ward at UCH, so that his psychological needs could be met as well as his physical ones. We were, if you like, writing the book as we went along, but it was about treating

> "Here I was again, trying to nurse someone in a completely inappropriate setting for their condition, because there was no appropriate place."

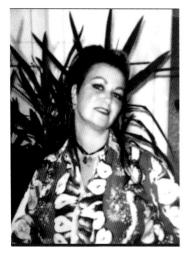

"It was a remarkable milestone in health care, and it changed the way we conduct palliative care."

"Many of my nursing colleagues, male and female, were gay themselves, as am I, and this helped drive through change quickly. It was a remarkable milestone in health care, and it changed the way we conduct palliative care."

people with respect and dignity, seeing the person as the primary point of care.

The fascinating aspect of HIV care for me is how much it was led by activism: gay men who were outraged by what was happening and how they were victimised and demonised, who shouted from the rooftops and demanded that the NHS and the drug companies took notice. Many of my nursing colleagues, male and female, were gay themselves, as am I, and this helped drive through change quickly. It was a remarkable milestone in health care, and it changed the way we conduct palliative care. I would argue that, funding cuts notwithstanding, the legacy of HIV is its revolutionary and lasting impact on our health service.

I began working at the London Lighthouse in 1994. I loved the place, a sympathetic setting where both physical and mental needs could be met. I was a charge nurse on the residential unit, dealing with people who presented with a broad spectrum of psychological problems, from understandable anxiety or depression about their situation through to HIV-related dementia and other psychoses. Some came in for regular respite to give carers a break, some needed a period of convalescence after hospital, and some were there because they were dying and needed as good a death as possible. I feel privileged to have sat, at their request, with dozens as they died, helping them feel safe enough to let go. The thought of some of those people still makes me cry.

Every time someone died, we would light a candle on the main reception desk, with a card by it with the person's name. You would know when you came into work to start your shift whether someone you'd been caring for had died overnight. It's a tradition I keep even now and, although I'm an atheist, I always open a window to let the person's spirit out, because when you are with someone as they die you can feel that moment of transition.

There was a mortuary at the Lighthouse so that families and friends could say last farewells, if they hadn't been there at the end. Some were still reeling from only discovering their son or brother was gay when they learned his diagnosis, and then that he was dying. Some families were wonderful, at the bedside for week after week until the end. We would be invited to funerals, but I rarely went. There were just too many to go to.

> "Some families were wonderful, at the bedside for week after week until the end. … though for some families, the rifts were irreconcilable."

We encouraged people to make living wills, which would not only cover how they wanted to be treated in their last hours, but also whom to call. I vividly remember one young man who had been outed as a very young teenager and thrown out of the family home by homophobic parents. In order to survive he became a rent boy. He was still only in his early twenties when we sat down with him to make his living will. He told us that under no circumstances, even if he no longer understood what was happening to him, should we call his mother.

Towards the end of his life, he developed dementia. As he lay dying, he began to cry for his mother, and begged us to call her. He had no recollection at all of the last fifteen years and the catastrophic row with his parents. He was terribly distressed, so we were faced with a dilemma. The living will was, to us, a morally binding document. He had been adamant before dementia set in that we should not call his mother, whatever happened, yet now he was a child again, desperate for her comfort. From everything he had told us, we were sure she wouldn't come. We consulted his friends and decided we should try to find his mother. It turned out she was wracked with guilt and distress about how she'd treated him, and she came to see him and hold him one last time before he died. It had been the right thing to do – though for some families, the rifts were irreconcilable.

When, a couple of years later, protease inhibitors like Ritonavir came on stream, I'm embarrassed to say I didn't hold out much hope; the side effects were horrendous, and many people were already too sick to gain any benefit. Some,

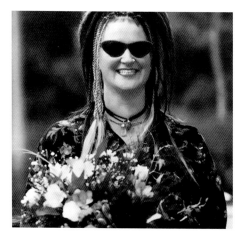

"But over the next two years, we began seeing a real change. Suddenly people were living with HIV. There were still hospitalisations, but people weren't dying in the numbers they had before."

like Efavirenz, even added to their mental health problems because they caused sleep disturbance and horrific nightmares indistinguishable from reality. But over the next two years, we began seeing a real change. Suddenly people were living with HIV. There were still hospitalisations, but people weren't dying in the numbers they had before. The residential unit at the Lighthouse closed because there was no longer a need for it, and I moved to a new job at the Kobler Clinic at the Chelsea and Westminster Hospital.

Mental health care was as important as ever for HIV patients. Some had lived so long in the expectation they were going to die that they now couldn't cope with surviving. They might feel guilt that antiretrovirals saved them, but had come too late to save a beloved friend or partner. Others got into trouble because they had incurred massive debts, in the expectation they would not be around when the bailiffs came to call, but now they had to pay it all back. Some couldn't work out if they wanted to live or die, and began playing Russian roulette with their medication, stopping it for weeks at a time then frantically going back to it. The apocalypse that had decimated social networks for so many gay people took its toll. There were issues with alcohol and party drugs, and a growing crystal meth problem associated with the gay scene, where people got so out of their heads, they were incapable of practising safe sex regardless of their HIV status – not to mention the associated paranoia and psychosis. The club drugs clinic I was instrumental in setting up was geared to specifically address those issues around sexual behaviour, chem sex and the gay scene.

"The apocalypse that had decimated social networks for so many gay people took its toll. ... The club drugs clinic I was instrumental in setting up was geared to specifically address those issues around sexual behaviour, chem sex and the gay scene."

I wish I could say everything is fine now, but people still die from AIDS – mostly those diagnosed late. There is still ignorance and prejudice about HIV. Not so long ago, I was chatting to a nurse who asked where I used to work. When I said I had looked after HIV patients for a large part of my working life, she was stunned. "Really? All that time? And you never caught it?" I thought back to how I'd tried to impress upon colleagues the importance of universal hygiene and precautions, whoever you look after. The person you know to be HIV positive is much less risk to you than the person who hasn't told you, or who doesn't know themselves. We need to tell these histories to a new generation, reminding them that although we have treatments, we still don't have a cure for HIV and AIDS.

"We need to tell these histories to a new generation, reminding them that although we have treatments, we still don't have a cure for HIV and AIDS."

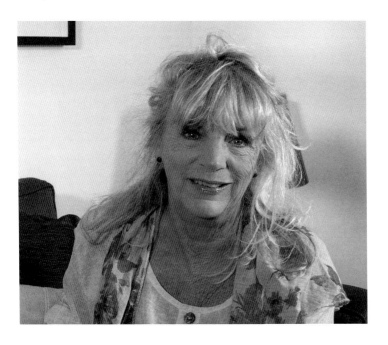

Adrienne Seed is an artist, writer and HIV campaigner, diagnosed with HIV/AIDS in 2002. She trained at St Martin's Art College, and spent many years living around the Mediterranean, painting, sculpting and running dance classes. After diagnosis, she returned to Lancashire, where she was born, and trained as a counsellor to equip herself with the skills to help others in her situation. For over ten years she has run an HIV website called HiVine and a support group in Blackburn for women and men with HIV.

Although her partner died of AIDS-related illness in 1998, Adrienne was not diagnosed herself until four years later, by which time she had a viral load of over 2 million. She found being a woman with HIV a lonely experience at first, and hid her status from her son for many years.

"I remember saying to my mother, "Mum, I'm HIV positive" – it was the first time I said those words – and she looked at me and said, "Don't worry, love, we can cope with this." Though it wasn't that easy."

Adrienne Seed
"I felt entirely on my own …"

It was 1998 when my partner died of liver cancer – or so I thought. He and I had been sailing around the Mediterranean together, and I was devastated when he died. Although I didn't know it at the time, very early in our relationship he'd had a brief fling with a Russian woman who must have been carrying the virus.

It wasn't long after his death that I started to feel unwell myself. It started with the kind of illness you get when you are run down: oral thrush, persistent cough, then rashes all over my body. I'd been working in Italy on some marble sculptures and suddenly my hands were so weak I found I couldn't lift them. Over the next four years, I became sicker and sicker. The family doctor kept doing tests but could find nothing obvious wrong. Then I went down with pneumonia while I was on Ibiza and was in hospital for two weeks. Although I had blood tests there every day, I was a straight, middle-aged white woman so no one thought to look for HIV. It was only when I consulted a homeopathic doctor on the island that he suspected immediately what was wrong. He sent off another blood test and broke the news to me three days later. When I came back to England to have the blood results reconfirmed at Blackburn Hospital, it turned out my viral load was over two million.

It was a terrible shock. Everything changes. You have to become a new person to deal with it. I remember saying to my mother, "Mum, I'm HIV positive" – it was the first time I said those words – and she looked at me and said, "Don't worry, love, we can cope with this." Though it wasn't that easy. For the first couple of years, I carried on getting one illness after another, including shingles so badly the hospital photographed them for their archives. My mother was elderly and arthritic, so at one stage we weren't sure who was caring for whom. If I had been diagnosed earlier, we wouldn't have had to go through that.

I was never angry with my partner for having passed the virus to me. We're all human, and he didn't know he was carrying it. But the medication I took made me hallucinate. I'd feel my feet turn into forks, or once I was a Mississippi riverboat, my hands in huge boxing gloves. That was hard, and I

"… one put his arm round me and said "Welcome to the club, love." It was so wonderful to be touched; until then I'd been paranoid about letting anyone near me."

only persevered by thinking of the pills as my little soldiers, marching through my body to kill the virus. The trippiness crept into my paintings, which have always been colourful and surrealistic. One, called *The Last Supper*, was my first attempt to portray how I felt. It shows me as Alice in Wonderland, alone at a table laid with empty bowls and enormous pills, while in the background men are carrying me away on a bier. Another shows a woman balancing on a tightrope, trying to reach the other side.

I didn't know any women who were HIV positive and felt entirely on my own. The only place I knew to go for support was George House Trust in Manchester. I found a group of gay men outside smoking, and when I sat down to join them one put his arm round me and said, "Welcome to the club, love." It was so wonderful to be touched; until then I'd been paranoid about letting anyone near me.

I didn't feel able to tell my son, who was in his twenties. It was only when I went for counselling after the death of my mother that I confessed how worried I was about accidentally infecting him – should I let him know? And the counsellor of course didn't tell me what to do, but gently put it to me that some would say Ben had a right to know. The idea began to churn in my brain until, one day, Ben and I were having an argument and I blurted out: "Stop it, you're making me ill!" He asked what was wrong with me. So I told him, and a huge weight lifted from my shoulders.

No one yet knows how HIV will affect people in their later years. What will it be like to be HIV positive in an old people's home? Because there is still a stigma attached. I won a free ticket for a facial massage a few years ago, but when I turned up at the beautician's she refused to treat me unless she wore rubber gloves. I tried to explain that my viral load is now undetectable and has been for years, so there is no way I can pass the virus on, but she insisted her insurance wouldn't allow it. I went home and cried because, once again, I was the great untouchable. And that's not the only example. I started going for walks with a male friend, and when we came back after walking our dogs one day, he found an unopened condom placed on the bonnet of his car, which I can only presume was one of my neighbours deciding to warn him that if he was thinking of starting a relationship with me, he'd better be careful.

> "Now there are more networks, so being diagnosed as a woman with HIV doesn't have to be the lonely experience I felt it was; it can be empowering."

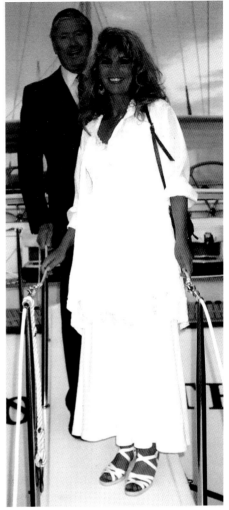

Adrienne with Brian on his yacht, 1995

Sadly, many women today still don't believe HIV is anything to do with them. It's still thought of as a gay man's disease, and I don't think it's widely understood that roughly half the people infected with HIV throughout the world are women. Now there are more networks, so being diagnosed as a woman with HIV doesn't have to be the lonely experience I felt it was; it can be empowering.

But though I can honestly say a lot of good things have come out of the last nineteen years, it still doesn't make up for what HIV took from me. Now my direction is always dictated by this thing inside me. It tried to kill me, and failed, but made me reliant on pills. It took the other me, the one that existed before the illness, when the world was full of possibility.

> "… roughly half the people infected with HIV throughout the world are women."

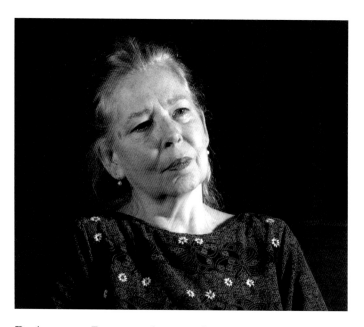

"All we wanted, as nurses, was to bring some sort of healing to our patients."

Barbara von Barsewisch trained as a nurse in London in the early 1990s and worked on Broderip Ward, the HIV ward at the Middlesex Hospital, for ten years. She went on to work at the Chelsea and Westminster Hospital in the Kobler Day Care Unit, where she developed an expertise in caring for patients with AIDS-related cancers, especially lymphomas. She now works as a clinical nurse specialist in haemato-oncology at the North Middlesex University Hospital NHS Trust. During the COVID-19 pandemic, she joined a bereavement support team reaching out to families who were not allowed to be with loved ones when they died in hospital.

"We couldn't cure them, but we felt our job was to offer at least an inner healing, so we did things we would never be able to do as nurses today. … I would never again have the courage to be so carefree, but like our patients we were young and brave then. "

Caring for patients with AIDS in the 1990s was a nursing experience unlike any other. It was a time when the rule book went out of the window and some extraordinary and moving interactions between nursing staff and patients helped to ease the passing of many of the people in Barbara's care.

Barbara von Barsewisch
"Some sort of healing…"

Thinking back to the 1990s, my mind conjures up endless lives, numerous men and women who I still carry within. Being asked to look back, three images stand out for me. These all happened on nightshifts. Night was the time on most wards when the telephone rarely rang, there were fewer distractions and everything seemed more intense…. One was of a tall, glamorous Italian man who came out of his room one night in a blue ballgown and six-inch heels before six-inch heels were commonplace. He looked so gorgeous as he sashayed towards the nursing station. Then he began to cough up lung tissue, dark, bloody flecks staining that beautiful blue gown.

Another is of a man close to the end of his life who was afraid of dying alone, rocking himself on his bed in pain because his back was covered with Kaposi's sarcoma and he couldn't lie down comfortably however tired he was. I sat with him, gently rubbing his back to ease it. He was so thin it felt as if I was touching a bird's skeleton.

A third was an African woman who was very religious. Every morning she asked the nurses to read to her from the Bible and prayer book by her bed. Then one day, she stopped asking. She was not far from death and, thinking it would comfort her, I asked her one night if she would like me to read from her Bible again. She said the illness was so terrible she had given up on God, since He had obviously given up on her. You can give someone pills for their pain, but how do you comfort someone who has lost their faith? I'm still troubled by that.

> "You can give someone pills for their pain, but how do you comfort someone who has lost their faith? I'm still troubled by that."

> "But AIDS was new and totally different – nobody had the answers. Everyone was learning at the same time, and we all had to work in partnership, something that changed doctor–patient interactions for good."

All we wanted, as nurses, was to bring some sort of healing to our patients. We couldn't cure them, but we felt our job was to offer at least an inner healing, so we did things we would never be able to do as nurses today. We didn't like the idea of a patient being discharged to a cold, empty flat, so for one patient a colleague and I jumped on a bus and beat the ambulance to his home to put on the heating. We made him a hot water bottle and tucked it in his bed, then returned to work. Those were the things we could do that made a difference. Another was when the comet Hale-Bopp was in the sky in 1997: during one night shift, when there was a clear wintry sky, a nurse who was doing the shift with me and I put patients into wheelchairs, wrapped them in blankets and took turns to take them out into Regent's Park to see the comet, a once-in-a-lifetime experience. We had such fun that night and the patients loved it. I could never do that now, and I would never again have the courage to be so carefree but, like our patients, we were young and brave then.

There was an extraordinary amount of laughter on Broderip Ward, usually over the tiny things in life because, suddenly, those tiny things really mattered. A cameo comes to mind from those days when I wasn't completely familiar with English idioms, so I remember giving a patient an intra-muscular injection, and instead of saying, as nurses usually do, you'll feel a sharp scratch, I said: "I'm sorry, I'm going to give you a small prick", and the entire ward erupted in laughter. I soon learned that wasn't the way to put it.

HIV/AIDS did change medical care in some respects. It had been quite paternalistic: the doctor had the answers and the patients did as they were told. But AIDS was new and totally different – nobody had the answers. Everyone was learning at the same time, and we all had to work in partnership, something that changed doctor–patient interactions for good. Patients have far more of a voice now than they did

"AIDS carried such a stigma that patients were often relieved when they received a cancer diagnosis. It meant they could admit they were ill: if they had cancer, people would pity them, but if they told the truth, that they had AIDS, they might be ostracised."

before HIV. It was also the advent of a real multi-disciplinary approach to care: all of a sudden dieticians, physios, social workers and others all became part of the patients' inpatient stay and discharge planning.

AIDS carried such a stigma that patients were often relieved when they received a cancer diagnosis. It meant they could admit they were ill: if they had cancer, people would pity them, but if they told the truth, that they had AIDS, they might be ostracised. The parents of one young man, who died of an AIDS-related chest infection, didn't want the words HIV or AIDS on the death certificate, which caused no end of difficulty. In the end we changed it to 'an antiretroviral complication', which fudged it enough for the parents, though anyone with an iota of medical knowledge would have understood what it meant. For that matter, my own parents would never admit to their neighbours I worked with HIV patients. They said I was on a cancer ward.

"So many of those young men had kept their London life secret from their parents."

So many of those young men had kept their London life secret from their parents. One patient asked us to contact his parents and invite them to the ward, but to say he had cancer – not entirely a lie, as he had an AIDS-related cancer. But when they arrived, it was obvious to them it was an HIV ward. They were elderly, and didn't understand anything about their son's lifestyle or the disease. The father didn't want to hold his son's hand, because he thought he could catch HIV from it – and if he showed any closeness to the boy, people watching might conclude he was a closet homosexual himself. The mother sat at the bedside apparently totally composed, clutching her handbag, and

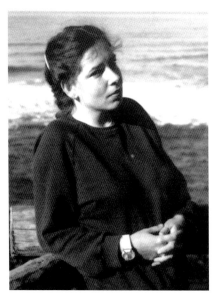

"That embodied for me what nursing could and should be – meeting a patient's needs in the most unexpected ways. The way we nursed those patients while they were dying is the best nursing the NHS has ever done, and I wish we could still do it that way."

didn't say a word, didn't touch him or speak to us, but she had the saddest eyes in the world. I will never forget her awful despair.

Some patients came back so frequently we knew them well. Oscar Moore was a journalist who wrote a column called PWA – Person with AIDS – for The *Guardian*, a witty, handsome man in his thirties who brought laughter and brightness to the ward. He was allowed onto the ward as a 'social' admission – something you would never find nowadays because the NHS is too stretched – admitted for a few nights for respite because he was finding it hard to cope at home. The next time he was with us, he asked if I had brought my bicycle onto the ward. I couldn't think what he meant until he pointed to the wheelchair by his bed. In just a few weeks, he had become so blind and confused he could no longer identify a wheelchair only a few feet away. His end was very quiet; he just slipped away on a whisper, breathed, then breathed no more.

I kept a diary and noted every time a patient died. After three years, there were more than 150 names of men and women on the list, almost one death a week.

One memory that sums up our approach to nursing in those years for me is Billy. He was older than most of our patients, 54, a tiny Scotsman who arrived on the ward with all his belongings in black bin liners, bags and bags of stuff, and a guitar. He loved music, and played his guitar all the time – we had to negotiate with other patients to let him play it. He'd found God at some point in what had been a difficult life, and religion was important to him but so was his music. As he became sicker, he played his guitar less and less. We moved him into a side room with all his bags and a radio, which another of the nurses, Lucy, would switch on for him, and he'd sit on his bed rocking and saying Jesus loves me, Jesus loves me, as if he needed to convince himself.

One Sunday afternoon, I came onto the ward to find Lucy carting black bags out of his room, piling them up by the nurse's station. Next, she pushed the bed out into the corridor, emptying Billy's room completely. Then she tuned the radio to a programme of dance music. She and Billy started to dance in his empty room, the waltz, the cha cha, the foxtrot. They were perfectly in harmony, completely at peace dancing together. That embodied for me what nursing could and should be – meeting a patient's needs in the most unexpected ways. The way we nursed those patients while they were dying is the best nursing the NHS has ever done, and I wish we could still do it that way.

"Soon, everything in HIV was pharmaceutically-driven. We more often saw people who were ill because of side-effects caused by their treatment, not because of AIDS."

Around 1996, the first anti-retroviral drugs arrived, and slowly the death rate began to fall. Soon, everything in HIV was pharmaceutically-driven. We more often saw people who were ill because of side-effects caused by their treatment, not because of AIDS. A large part of our job was to motivate patients to remain on their medication. Western people with HIV were generally open to trying the drugs, whereas many African patients were much more reluctant, fatalistic about letting AIDS kill them. Eventually fewer beds were needed, so Broderip Ward closed and we were moved to another part of the hospital. I used to go up to Broderip to look into the empty ward and remember the patients I'd met. One day, a man had beaten me to it, peering through the doors, the partner of a patient who'd died, there to remember too.

"Nurses are important to patients, but the reverse is also true – we remember patients and are shaped by them. I'm a different person, and a better nurse, because of all the people I've nursed into death, and I still feel the loss of those young men and women. And if I feel like this all these years on, how must their family, friends and partners feel?"

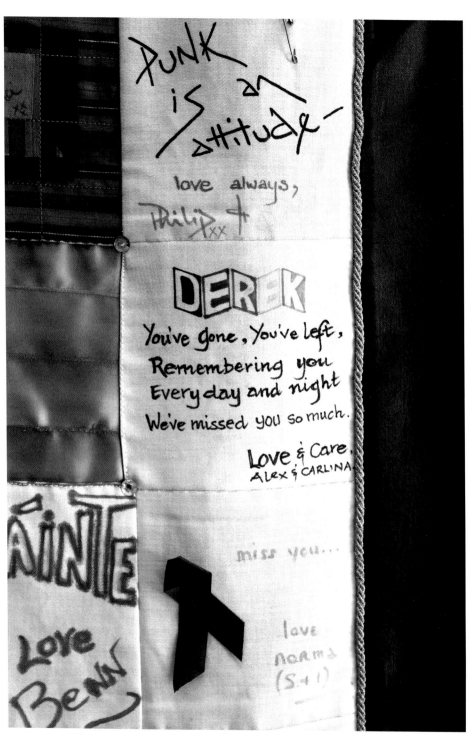

Detail from one of the quilt panels, collected by the AIDS Memorial Quilt Preservation Partnership.

Part III:
2000–the present

In July 2000, the Joint United Nations Programme on HIV/AIDS (UNAIDS) negotiated with five pharmaceutical companies to reduce antiretroviral drug prices in developing countries. In June 2001, the United Nations (UN) General Assembly called for the creation of a "global fund" to support efforts by countries and organisations towards ending AIDS through prevention, treatment and care. In November, the World Trade Organization (WTO) announced the Doha Declaration which allowed developing countries to manufacture generic medications in response to public health crises, like the AIDS pandemic.

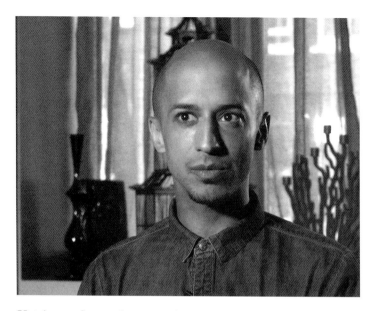

Krishen Samuel was born in Johannesburg, South Africa in 1986. He studied Speech-Language Pathology at university in Cape Town, then came to London in 2016 to study for a master's degree in Global Health Public Health and Policy. He has written for *The Huffington Post* UK on HIV/AIDS and LGBTQ issues, and is currently doing his PhD in Public Health on a Fulbright scholarship in the US.

"... during the 1980s and 1990s, the country lost sight of the AIDS epidemic as it slowly took hold. ...By the end of the 1990s, the situation was desperate. People were dying daily."

"Because HIV in South Africa was surrounded by stigma and discrimination, it was hard to open the right conversations, even within the gay community."

Krishen Samuel was not even born when the AIDS pandemic began, but he grew up in a country which has seen some of the highest infection rates for HIV in the world. Since being diagnosed with HIV in 2009, he has become aware of the need to communicate his experience and not forget what happened in the 1980s and 1990s.

Krishen Samuel
"All those who came before me, that's part of my story."

For a country which traditionally had quite conservative, religious ideals, South Africa is surprisingly progressive, especially in terms of gay rights – perhaps because gay people played an important part in the struggle against apartheid. We are the only African country to allow gay marriage and gay adoption.

However, because of the political changes happening in South Africa during the 1980s and 1990s, the country lost sight of the AIDS epidemic as it slowly took hold. AIDS was not spoken about openly, which may explain why it has inflicted such a huge toll on South Africa, with one of the highest infection rates in the world. By the end of the 1990s, the situation was desperate. People were dying daily. Many children were orphaned, many were left homeless, grandparents stepping in because both parents had died, and many children were themselves HIV positive. Perhaps a domestic worker might go home to the rural areas and never come back, and it would be whispered by her employers that she had AIDS, but it wasn't seen as a white, middle-class condition, it was deemed a condition that affected poorer black people on the fringes of society.

For a long time, the government was in denial that people living with HIV needed access to medication. It was only in the early 2000s, much later than in the UK and the US, after the Treatment Action Campaign organised protests and marches, that people could get the drugs they needed through the public health system.

When I went to university in Cape Town, away from home, I saw it as a wonderful opportunity to explore my sexuality in a famously gay city. My course was taught on the medical campus so we were given lectures about the dangers of contracting HIV through sexual activity. A woman came in to talk about her experience of living with HIV, bringing along all her medication, eight or more pills a day. That gave me pause for thought. I was terrified afterwards of becoming infected and always at the back of my mind was a voice shrieking: *I hope I don't get it! I hope I don't get it!* Because the condition in South

"It's a watershed moment, because you know you can never turn back the clock and be the person you were before."

Africa was surrounded by stigma and discrimination, it was hard to open the right conversations, even within the gay community. How and when do you ask a new partner about their HIV status? How do you negotiate condom use? Being so paranoid, I did get myself tested regularly: in 2008, I had eight tests, all negative. Every time, I went through the same harrowing process, realising I'd slipped up, going for a test, the anxiety as I waited for results, then a huge sigh of relief.

The following year my anxiety abated a little, so I had few qualms when I had a routine medical screening. A few days later, the doctor's office called to tell me there was a small problem with my white blood cell count. When I went in to see the doctor, she hadn't had a chance to go through my results, and was reading them as I sat there. She turned a page, and her face fell. "You're HIV positive." The room started to spin. I couldn't focus on what she said after that. It's a watershed moment, because you know you can never turn back the clock and be the person you were before.

These days, with drugs that can hold the condition at bay, we often compare HIV to diabetes or other long term, chronic illnesses. But it doesn't feel like that when you get the diagnosis. For me, it was like having to come out to my family all over again – but *worse* than coming out, because it felt more shameful. I kept berating myself: how could I have been so stupid, knowing HIV was a huge problem in my country? How could I have let myself become infected?

My sister managed to change the way I was thinking, by saying: "You're a sexually active young man, you live in a country with one of the highest infection rates in the world. Don't take it so personally! Think of it as living in a war zone and being hit by a stray bullet. This isn't the end of your story, you're not going to die."

Reframing it like that was empowering. It helped me step back and stop blaming myself, and consider instead how I would manage the condition. Because my CD4 count had not yet fallen below 200, the level at which treatment was then deemed necessary, I didn't start immediately on medication, but my viral load was monitored and I started treatment eight months later. Meanwhile, I used the Internet to find and contact someone who'd lived with HIV for 25 years, which helped reassure me. Medically, there have been amazing advances to keep the viral load in check. Now mine is undetectable, which means I can't pass on the virus.

In South Africa, only my family and a few close friends knew I was positive. But when I came to London to study for my master's degree, it seemed an opportunity to reinvent myself and be more open. I joined a group called Youth Stop AIDS, a campaigning organisation active on university campuses. The group's slogan is "It ain't over," and they are passionate about people getting tested and accessing treatment. It's not the HIV+ person on medication, and therefore undetectable, that should be feared, it's the person who hasn't been tested and doesn't yet know they have it.

In the UK, there is complacency, even denial, over HIV, and young people often assume AIDS is a condition of the past, something that happened in the 1980s. Amazingly, the others on my course, studying for a postgraduate degree in global health, didn't think of HIV as close to home. Straight friends would say they only used condoms to prevent pregnancy. Even if they did consider sexually transmitted infections, HIV was far down the list of those they imagined being exposed to.

The UK has been one of the biggest funders globally for HIV and AIDS related programmes, but now AIDS is slipping lower and lower on the agenda for the UK government, although there are still parts of the world where, every day, people die of AIDS. The minute we assume it's over is the moment it will start creeping back.

Looking back at the 1980s and 1990s, I feel touched by all those lives that were lost. For me, as a gay man who is HIV positive, those who came before me are part of my story too. As a community we still carry the battle scars, and the unpleasant parts of the gay experience should not be whitewashed. Never forget those who died, because their stories are part of the history that binds us and takes us forward into the future.

> "It's not the HIV+ person on medication … that should be feared, it's the person who hasn't been tested and doesn't yet know they have it."

> "In the UK, there is complacency, even denial, over HIV, and young people often assume AIDS is a condition of the past."

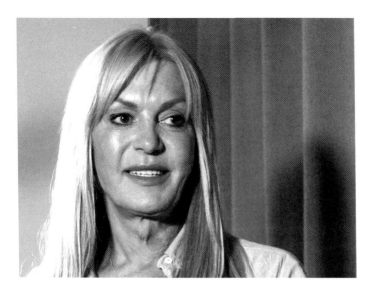

"With addiction, you need to hit rock bottom before you can change, but for me there always seemed to be further depths to plumb."

Rebecca de Havilland is a trans woman born in Ireland, who had a successful career as a hair and make-up artist in Dublin and ran a model agency before moving to London and seeking gender reassignment surgery after a failed marriage. She has volunteered with the Terrence Higgins Trust and now project-manages the 56T service for trans and non-binary people in London. She also runs her own Project Bootcamp to support trans women through the transitioning process.

"When I finally told my daughter I was HIV positive, she said that she loved me and was proud of me… ."

It was only when Rebecca applied for gender-reassignment surgery that she discovered she was HIV positive. Her journey through HIV and AIDS has been a journey into understanding herself. Working as an escort to earn money for the operation, she became addicted to alcohol and drugs, but eventually managed to get her life back on track. After many years of trying to hide her HIV status from the world, she now talks openly about it and spreads the message that HIV and AIDS still pose a risk to young people having unprotected sex.

Rebecca de Havilland
"I was in denial about my illness."

From a very young age, I knew I was trapped in the wrong body, but Ireland then was a very conservative Catholic society and I didn't realise I could do anything about it. Fortunately, the 1970s were a wonderfully gender-fluid time to be growing up. Everyone had long hair and everyone wore flared jeans, platform shoes and make-up, emulating David Bowie and glam rock on the TV.

The word 'gay' wasn't used in Ireland then, you were 'queer'. People described me as 'light on my feet', which meant effeminate. Even Elton John hadn't come out then, so no one really talked about it. At 18, I bowed to the pressure to have a girlfriend. By now I knew it was possible to change sex – I'd heard of Caroline Cossey, a transexual model for *Vogue* and a Bond girl – but I wasn't going to divulge to anyone that I wanted to be a woman, or that I was attracted to men. I tried to persuade myself I was just going through a phase and thought getting married would fix everything. In all fairness, my mother knew I was making a mistake and did try and stop me, but quite how the rest of my family didn't work it out, I have no idea. I picked the wedding dress, and the bridesmaids' dresses!

In 1980 my daughter was born, and my career as a hairdresser was beginning to take off. Within two years I had a job in the top hair salon in Dublin, and styling for fashion shows and photo shoots. At the pinnacle, I did hair and make up for Johnny Logan at the Eurovision Song Contest, the year he won it in Belgium: I was

> "I tried to persuade myself I was just going through a phase and thought getting married would fix everything."

> "I was famous and sought-after. But inside I was suicidal."

111

"I came out as gay in a very colourful rainbow in 1983, but sex with men felt as uncomfortable as sex with women. I didn't seem to fit anywhere."

"They told me I couldn't have the operation and I had maybe two years to live. My whole world collapsed."

famous and sought-after. But inside I was suicidal. I had confided in my wife I was attracted to men; she threw me out and stopped me seeing my daughter, which broke my heart. I came out as gay in a very colourful rainbow in 1983, but sex with men felt as uncomfortable as sex with women. I didn't seem to fit anywhere.

I moved to London to further my career, discovered burlesque and drag at Madame JoJos, met trans women and, for the first time, understood who I really was. Eventually, I began the process of transitioning, taking hormones and getting approval from three psychiatrists. At that time, it was necessary to be tested for HIV before the surgery. It didn't occur to me for a moment that I might have the virus; I thought whoever's up there couldn't be that cruel.

When I was called into the room for my results, I knew immediately there was something wrong. They told me I couldn't have the operation and I had maybe two years to live. My whole world collapsed.

My family in Ireland couldn't cope and it drove a wedge between us. I remember overhearing one of my relatives say: "God, he would do anything for attention." At the time I was too selfishly bound up with myself to understand what a huge shock it was for them, and I was angry they weren't more supportive.

There used to be an unfunny joke doing the rounds that if AIDS doesn't kill you, the meds will. I was on AZT for a while and watched friends die, but couldn't bring myself to tell them I too had HIV. I'd lost my career, afraid to go back to Dublin, I was broke, living in London as a woman, and the only way I could raise money for surgery was to become a high-class escort. After the operation in 1991, I looked fabulous, but the clothes and handbags cost money, so I began doing 'extras', discovering that if I drank or drugged, it numbed me enough not to care what I did. I even ran a brothel in Amsterdam for a while, but champagne and cocaine gave way to crack and heroin and I was working the streets, doing twenty quid tricks down alleyways in Soho. My family thought I was dead, because I couldn't face going back to Ireland, ashamed of the mess I'd made of my life. I had zero self-respect, and very little memory of the next five years. I was skinny and gaunt, but people assumed it was my addiction. I remember catching sight of myself reflected in a shop window and thought it was some raddled old witch sneaking onto my patch to steal my punters.

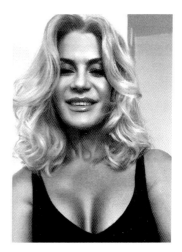

For a while, I was on combination therapy, but the meds had to be kept in a fridge and I didn't want anyone I shared a flat with to know I had HIV, so I stopped taking them. Every so often I would stagger into a clinic to get cleaned up and go on medication again. For a while, all would be well, then the whole sorry cycle would start over. With addiction, you need to hit rock bottom before you can change but, for me, there always seemed to be further depths to plumb. When I woke one morning on the floor with one broken hand and a bottle of vodka in the other, and no idea how I'd got there, I thought I'd hit the bottom and took myself to Alcoholics Anonymous. But I was wrong. I managed six months sober, then just couldn't do it anymore. I bought a half bottle of vodka, swallowed it along with handfuls of anti-depressant tablets and texted a friend for help. I woke two days later on a life-support machine in hospital. No sooner was I out, than I tried to buy another bottle of vodka and finish the job, but this time I was sectioned and committed to a mental hospital. That, finally, was rock bottom.

Only then did I grasp that the AA programme requires not just sobriety but honesty. You take a

> "I began doing 'extras', discovering that if I drank or drugged, it numbed me enough not to care what I did … champagne and cocaine gave way to crack and heroin and I was working the streets…"

113

> "... requires not just sobriety but honesty. You take a long hard look at yourself. I realised I'd blamed anyone else ... I went back to meetings and haven't touched a drink or a drug since. I was in denial about HIV even to myself. I thought the truth would lose me my newly discovered family."

long hard look at yourself. I realised I'd blamed anyone else for all that happened, instead of acknowledging my own part. I went back to meetings and haven't touched a drink or a drug since.

What happened next is almost like a fairy story. I re-established contact with my sister, went back to Ireland and met old friends who were opening a burlesque nightclub, where I then worked as Lady V on stage, looking like Big Bird, feathers coming out of everywhere. By an extraordinary coincidence, one night I discovered that my daughter, whom I hadn't seen since she was a child, worked there selling tickets. We were reunited and I met my granddaughter.

It seemed a happy ending, but although I then started a successful model agency in Ireland and published my life story, I had one more problem to conquer: I still wasn't able to be honest about my illness. I was in denial about HIV even to myself. I thought the truth would lose me my newly discovered family. I ran out of medication, and thought I must be safe to stop taking it since my last viral load test had shown I was down to undetectable levels. For almost a year, I ignored the signs: my hair fell out, my teeth were rotting, I was painfully thin and plagued with kidney infections. Eventually I was hospitalised with pneumonia in Dublin and told I had six months to live.

But after everything I'd been through, I refused to accept it would end like this. I sought a second opinion in London and was put on a clinical trial for some new AIDS medication. That summer was hell. I was living on benefits in bed-and-breakfast accommodation, I wore a wig, I had to have all my teeth removed, the meds didn't seem to be having any effect, and I knew I had only myself to blame for it all. But slowly, slowly over the next two years I began to improve. I promised myself that if I could reach undetectable levels of virus again, I would completely change my lifestyle.

At Christmas 2015, my viral load test showed undetectable. I signed up for the Back To Work programme at the Terrence Higgins Trust, trained in sexual health, and began volunteering with Positive Voices, which educates young people about HIV. When I finally told my daughter I was HIV positive, she said that she loved me and was proud of me: "Go and shout it from the rooftops."

I've been asked, now you've come out about having HIV, how do people treat you? I joke that they still run, but not as fast. But as I say to people – if you saw me walking down the street, would you think in a million years I have HIV? They say no – I look pretty good for a woman in her sixties. And then the penny drops. They realise you can't tell who has the virus and who hasn't. It could be your new boyfriend, your girlfriend. Anyone can be infected.

"And then the penny drops. They realise you can't tell who has the virus and who hasn't. it could be your new boyfriend, your girlfriend. Anyone can be infected."

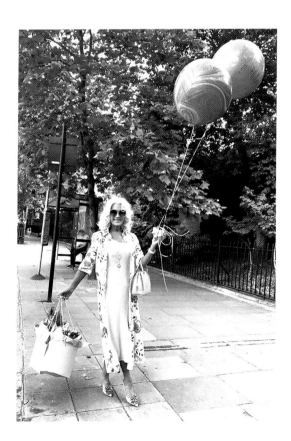

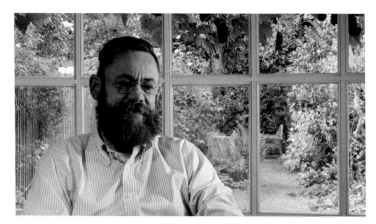

"Social pressures are potent triggers for mental illness."

Dr Rupert Whitaker holds a unique position in the history of HIV/AIDS – infected in 1981, he is one of the longest survivors with HIV and, with fourteen years' clinical and scientific training and using his own experiences as a patient, he has dedicated most of the past four decades to advocacy in medicine and public health for the benefit of people with HIV and, latterly, people with chronic conditions.

During a gap year in 1980 between school and university he went to Germany where he began a relationship with his first boyfriend and, by 1981, had fallen sick with an undiagnosable condition; physicians could only tell him there was a problem with his white blood cells. Returning to the UK to take up a university place, he met Terry Higgins and they became boyfriends. After Terry died from AIDS in 1982, Rupert and a few of Terry's friends decided to create the Terry Higgins Trust (which later became known as the Terrence Higgins Trust) in his memory. Rupert remained a trustee of the charity after moving to North America; there he studied psychiatry, neurology, and immunology, focusing on HIV, and took up various post-doctoral fellowships until he he had a stroke and was diagnosed with AIDS when he was thirty, ending his academic career. He is now an international expert witness in psychiatry and public health, a Fellow at the National Institute for Health and Care Excellence, and the founder and chairman of the Tuke Institute, an independent think-tank aiming to redesign medical services for the benefit of patients first and foremost. In 2021, he received an honorary degree of Doctor of Science for his services to medical science and patient-advocacy.

This piece focuses on Rupert's views on living long term with HIV, and his belief the LGBT-community needs to rally round once again to do more for the vulnerable while also reforming the model of medical services.

Rupert Whitaker
"Some of us are just surviving, not living …"

A t the time Terry died, we knew very little about the illness that was causing such a stir in America, which was called at the time 'Gay Related Immune Deficiency', or GRID. But we knew that if it was spreading in the LGBT-community in America, then Terry's death was proof that it would soon be spreading in the UK too. By then I was also too sick even to climb the two flights of stairs to the flat I lived in; a year after his death, Terry's physicians were surprised to find I was still alive.

Through the Terrence Higgins Trust, we were trying to organise and get ahead of the curve to prepare for the onslaught of what came to be known as AIDS. What we weren't prepared for was the degree of resistance from physicians, who felt they didn't need any help. Yet all they had to show for their self-sufficiency in the early days of the pandemic was a desperate scramble to try to stop people dying so quickly from a range of bizarre opportunistic diseases few had encountered before. Much of the rest of the actual care was provided by the community, going into homes and hospitals to work within the clinics and on the wards. Activism had a major effect on the nature of the response. In the US, for example, this included working with governmental scientists, drug-companies and federal officials to speed through the development of new medication, even changing the way clinical trials were conceptualised and carried out. But that very success ironically sowed seeds of future failure: once effective medication came out in 1996, physicians took back control; their view was the community was no longer needed in the clinics as now there were medications to treat the

"… we are still struggling to create a response to problems of mental illness, chronic disability, unemploy-ability, and ageing in the older cohort living with HIV."

> "Yes, we may now live an almost normal lifespan with HIV – but we do not necessarily live it well."

> "…that generation has been traumatised and some suffer from a kind of survivor-syndrome, a type of complex Post-Traumatic-Stress Disorder."

virus, regardless of the disabling and sometimes life-threatening toxicities they brought with them.

The consequence is that we are still struggling to create a response to problems of mental illness, chronic disability, unemployability, and ageing in the older cohort living with HIV, not to mention pervasive problems like chemsex across all age-groups with HIV and at risk of HIV-infection. The marvellous medications have stopped people dying but have also left a generation disabled rather than returned to health, while mental and social problems are sidelined. Meanwhile, problems with homophobia and transphobia remain to cause mental illness in affected youth, increasing their risk of HIV, substance-abuse, self-harm and so on, over time. "Health"-services' wilful blindness to these problems will not make them go away; they simply store them up for the future.

Yes, we may now live an almost normal lifespan with HIV – but we do not necessarily live it well. As we get older, we suffer disproportionately more from age-related illnesses, particularly the first generation of us for whom HIV-medications were not as well-developed as they are now, causing higher rates of heart-disease, dementia, arthritis, diabetes and so on. There are people whose lives have been wrecked by HIV, who have been on disability and welfare for decades, if they haven't been thrown off it through the government's hostile environment towards the disabled. Some of us are only surviving, not living.

We need to look at housing and find care and accommodation for those who have no family to look after them in old age. Again, we need to look at mental illness. A generation of people were affected by HIV and AIDS – not only those of us with the virus, but also those who had to live alongside it, wiping up their lover's vomit as he died; that generation has been traumatised and some suffer from a kind of survivor-syndrome, a type of complex Post Traumatic Stress Disorder. That's about personal loss and the stress that comes from living long term under the threat that either you, or people close to you, will die. Often – and I can speak personally here – it manifests as what the sufferer imagines is a self-sufficiency, but which is actually withdrawal and detachment. You cannot continually be saturated with grief and stress for so many years without finding a way to stop yourself feeling so inexpressibly raw, to cope with wounds that haven't been allowed to heal. Most everyone can get over a broken heart or two in the course of their life. But thirty? Forty? Learning how to trust that you can rely on someone, that they are not going to die too soon, is hard. It becomes difficult to form new relationships and it isolates. If you do try to reconnect, there are volatile feelings, distress and anger, the desire to be able to walk away at any point, which doesn't make for healthy relationships. Over time, this becomes normal, so that people enter lives of everyday misery and become unable to imagine anything better.

Many of us have been through this, but we rarely talk about it. Instead, we have a sense of fear of the future in all its manifestations. How will you work out what is normal illness when you are getting old or what is a toxic effect of the medications on your already-damaged body? You can see a lot of problematic self-care that turns into self-harm, people managing by misusing alcohol, drugs, or sex that isn't healthy. Survivors killed themselves because they could no longer bear the pain of surviving so many losses, including the final one, the loss of a community with a shared purpose.

Social pressures are potent triggers for mental illness. Losing your disability-welfare, or becoming isolated long-term because you are shielding through lockdowns, such things can reactivate old trauma. You can lose your courage and will to fight through the day — and being disabled often requires fighting through the day. Remarkable as the new drugs are, research I carried out identified a telling problem: the greater the loss you suffered through HIV, the more friends who died, the less likely you are to take your meds today, no matter how long you have been infected. You will also be more likely to have arguments with your physician or disengage from services. It's a form of self-harm, fostered by medical services that are wilfully blind to the importance of mental and social issues.

> "Learning how to trust that you can rely on someone, that they are not going to die too soon, is hard."

> "Instead, we have a sense of fear of the future …"

"A major issue … is that neither social nor mental issues are addressed adequately by clinics."

"… sexual infections now are the worst since the Second World War."

A major issue, not just for long term HIV survivors but all people with HIV or at risk of it, is that neither social nor mental issues are addressed adequately by clinics. Within the NHS, everything is compartmentalised and physical illness and mental illness are dealt with in different silos. The only reason for this is because it works for physicians, who believe that only they do 'real' (i.e., physical) medicine; what is best for the patient is considered only secondarily to that. The integrated teams we saw in the early days of the HIV pandemic no longer exist. Yes, your physician might assess you and refer you to mental health services, but is that different from a social worker determining whether or not you need a referral to oncology because you have a suspicious lump? The presenting problem is not within the physician's competency (regardless of what they claim), nor the social worker's, so why do we allow the first if not the second?

The problem with a physician-centred approach is that it becomes: *We have a pill for that!* For example, take pre-exposure prophylaxis (PrEP) against HIV-infection. When someone turns up in a clinic saying they're worried about the risk of contracting HIV, because they're having sex without condoms, it's not enough simply to offer them PrEP. Why are they not having safer sex? As HIV-infections have gone down over the past ten years, syphilis has become epidemic; ditto with gonorrhoea etc.; sexual infections now are the worst since the Second World War. Is that person at the clinic also using harder recreational drugs to have sex, which can indicate mental illness, particularly anxiety, depression, and substance-dependencies? Are they feeling lonely and isolated? These factors are all potent predictors of illness. With the wrong clinicians not asking the right questions, it's obvious that we should set person-centred standards for medical services, so that they're not just about our bodies, but competently addressing our physical, mental, and social health all together. Similarly, we need to audit clinics in a way that isn't just a review of how many blood tests they do, how many infections they diagnose, but how are they really helping people to get well — and stay well? Some of the help can only come from the community, not clinical

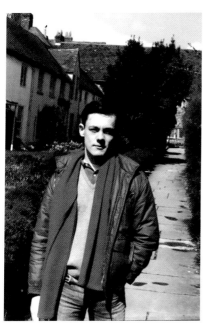

"Some of the help can only come from the community, not clinical health services on their own, but our excellent model for that not only didn't develop further, it was wiped out."

health services on their own, but our excellent model for that not only didn't develop further, it was wiped out. We need to answer "who benefits from that?" and change that fact.

As a young man, barely a decade after the legalisation of homosexual acts in the UK, I saw a true LGBT-community emerging, bonded by a common fight against bigotry; with AIDS, that community came together with a vengeance. Change only occurs if you really push — often only if you stand up and shout. It should be recognised that the LGBT-community and our allies radically changed the face of the response to the HIV-pandemic. We should be very proud of that. We learned lessons for how to respond effectively to a pandemic; those lessons were forgotten in Covid. We showed how to create fundamental changes in our health-services too, so that they became about people and health, not just bodies and disease, creating a model of how to treat all people with chronic conditions effectively. That lesson has also been forgotten, the model wiped out.

"This is not good enough. For the community of people living with HIV, particularly long-term survivors, people with complex comorbidities, and the ageing, it's time to get ahead of the curve again."

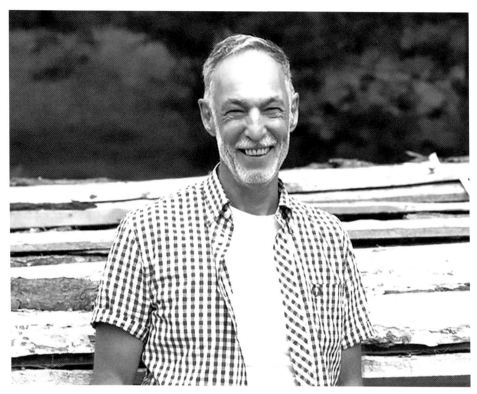

"In my early 40s I was dauntless, I had a brilliant career, a beautiful partner, I had friends and we were all doing so well. And then, in the blink of an eye, it stopped…"

Earlier in the book we heard from David Eason describing the personal impact of AIDS during the 1980s and 1990s when so many of his friends died. This account covers what happened to David, himself diagnosed as HIV positive, after his partner died, and how HIV continues to affect his life today.

"But against all sense, I kept returning to the thought – I can hardly even say it was a hope – that maybe, just maybe, I would get through it, and be able to say one day that 'I lived through the age of AIDS.'"

David Eason – Part II
"Coping ..."

At one point after my partner Gary died, someone asked me: "How are you coping?" All I could say was: "I have no idea." It's like standing on a hill top with an enormous wind buffeting you, yet somehow blowing straight through you, because there are huge gaps inside. Some of the pieces of you as a person are missing; others are shattered and are in pieces on the floor. Gary and I had been living on air for months, poor as church mice because I'd lost my business, we'd sold our flat to pay the debts, and we were completely preoccupied with Gary's illness. Some days it was a case of either eating or taking the tube to the hospital, because I couldn't afford to do both. Then suddenly he was gone, and all that changed because his life insurance policy paid up, his employer Virgin Atlantic honoured his death in service benefit and, for the first time in months, I didn't have to worry about money. But that was all I had. AIDS had taken everything and everyone else. One person remained alive in the UK, my old friend Neil whose own partner Bill died six months before Gary, so I stayed with him for a while, both of us shocked and numb as we tried to think of what was next?

I didn't know how long I had to live, either. When I tested positive in 1990, the doctor had told me I probably had six or seven years left. But against all sense, I kept returning to the thought – I can hardly even say it was a hope – that maybe, just maybe I would get through it, and be able to say one day that "I lived through the age of AIDS."

But since I now had money, but no home or friends, I decided to travel – or perhaps a more accurate word would

> "But that was all I had. AIDS had taken everything and everyone else."

"All the time, I was half-looking for a new home, a new life, a big strong man to take me in his arms and make it all right again, yet at the same time, secretly, I knew I could never allow anyone to take away that pain that had come so hard earned."

"We wanted a space where we could build a tribe supportive of the positive community. "

be run. I ran and ran and ran for almost a year. Because Gary had worked for Virgin, Richard Branson was generous and gave me a number of free tickets to fly wherever I wanted. I went to Mardi Gras in Sydney, because Gary and I had wanted to do that together but couldn't afford it while he was alive. From there I went on to New Zealand. All the time, I was half-looking for a new home, a new life, a big strong man to take me in his arms and make it all right again, yet at the same time, secretly, I knew I could never allow anyone to take away that pain that had come so hard earned.

When I eventually stopped running and with nowhere else to go, I came back to London, I met Spike Rhodes and Dominic Gough who were involved in a magazine called *Positive Nation*, for HIV positive people. I began writing articles with them, and together we also became involved in a venture to trial a gay radio station for a while. It was from our exploits in "The Positive Zone" on "Freedom FM" that we decided that what was needed was a club-night, specifically aimed at positive people. At that time, 1995/1996, within the gay community itself there was a lot of discrimination and people didn't talk about being HIV positive, not if you didn't want everyone to leave the room.… We were the exception, all widows and open about our status. We wanted a space where we could build a tribe supportive of the positive community. We had no idea really how to run a club-night but we were seasoned clubbers so how hard could it be? Initially everyone thought we were crazy, but we found a backer, John Newman at Turnmills, a very famous London venue, who liked our idea and gave us the Sunday night slot, but instead of a monthly club he wanted it every week. We were overwhelmed and ecstatic. We called it 'Warriors'. It became astonishingly successful, with sometimes a crowd of a thousand people

"We called it 'Warriors'. It became astonishingly successful …

turning up. Sometimes people would arrive visibly unwell, some with their faces covered in Kaposi's sarcoma, just to forget everything and have one last dance. They came supported by their friends and carrying their meds which we'd store behind the till for them. Everyone was supportive of each other and it was a remarkable place. Any profit we made went to Food Chain, a charity providing hot meals for housebound people living with AIDS. Because I looked after the business side of things, once the tills were set up, etc., I didn't have anything else to do until the end of the night, but after a while it became obvious to me that I did have an informal but crucial role. I would be walking around being visible and chatting to people enjoying themselves, and once I was approached by a young guy, who asked if he could have a quiet word. We went up to the coffee shop and he suddenly disclosed that he was 18 years old and he'd been diagnosed two weeks ago, and was terrified his life was over and there was no-one he could really talk to. Yet here was an elder, an HIV positive man, running a club-night, unafraid – a role model! Afterwards this happened quite often and I realised that I was becoming a kind of informal club counsellor, someone to turn to in a non-medical setting, someone like them, and I've continued in that ever since.

I was lucky in that throughout those years I remained healthy but, eventually, in 2002, I started to become ill. Suddenly my face in the mirror was pale and gaunt; I felt cold all the time. I knew I didn't have any kind of a future; I was going to become sicker and all I could think was there was no purpose in carrying on or starting to take medication: when you've lost so much, what's the frigging point? But a friend gave me a reality check: "You need to decide whether you

> "Everyone was supportive of each other and it was a remarkable place. Any profit we made went to Food Chain, a charity providing hot meals for housebound people living with AIDS."

"…in 2002, I started to become ill. … But a friend gave me a reality check: 'You need to decide whether you are ready to go, or whether you want to stay?' I decided to stay. Before long the medication began to work …"

are ready to go, or whether you want to stay?" I decided to stay. Before long the medication began to work, which gave me the impetus to start trying to heal myself emotionally as well. In 2005 I met a new partner, Matt, and realised I could live again. He supported me in so many ways including paying for the Kinesiology and Healing courses that enabled me to earn again and have a purpose again. He gave me my life back. By 2009 I recognised I had done all I could for my friends but there was another step I needed to take. It's impossible to live a life carrying all those thoughts, all that pain, all those memories, all that history. Eventually I had to let them go and I performed a little ceremony to honour them and let them go forever. There's no dishonour in not celebrating all those birthdays and those death days. You celebrate life by living it.

But those of us who came through those years don't fit easily with the world. It's impossible to talk to people who haven't been through what you've experienced, and hope for any kind of deep connection or understanding. We are a generation of gay men who never expected to get old, but now we *are* getting old. The medication has worked for us and we are no longer dying *en masse*, but there are long term effects we don't yet understand. We often don't have families to care for us if we get ill. A few years ago, a man I'd met while volunteering, died in a hospice. A friend asked me to go to the funeral. When we arrived at the crematorium there was no plan, no flowers, no music, just two people from the men's group and a couple of gay neighbours. Between us we improvised a little eulogy and organised some music and bid him farewell; by now we were really good at funerals. And maybe that will be happening more and more as this generation of gay men grows old. Perhaps we need to come together again and organise the way we did during the AIDS pandemic, build gay retirement homes and start other new projects.

I think one of the great losses from AIDS is that we lost a generation of teachers and talented people, who would now be in their 60s and 70s and could have helped the next generation deal with their sexuality. Gay men today in particular are suffering as a result of that, because they have had fewer heroes, role models and mentors to look to.

"You can lose everything but, if you have hope, you have a chance. Losing hope, you lose yourself. That so nearly happened to me but somehow, I held on."

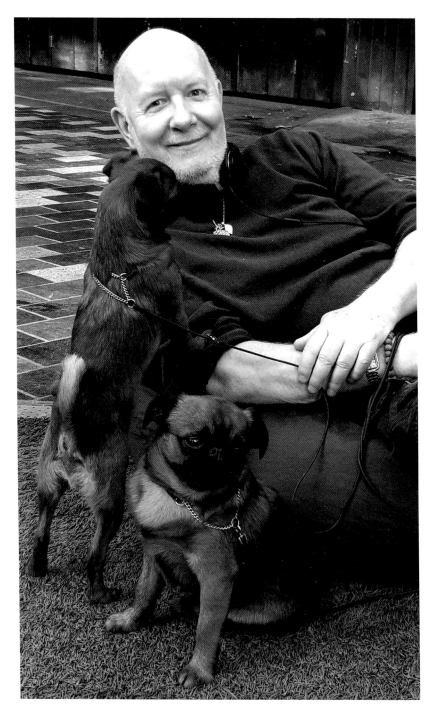

We heard earlier on in this book how George Hodson managed to survive from HIV after losing his partner, business and many friends. Here George reflects on his life today, the cost of survival and a future that has many challenges.

George Hodson - Part II
"My sleeping dragon …"

My biggest challenge now is to how to survive the chronic poverty I've been forced into by being unable to work. I have no savings and I live on benefits, so I'm scared my poverty leaves me no real choices as I age. I've survived three cancers and a heart bypass operation and I'm weary, I've done a lot of fighting. The thing I fear most is being shuffled off into a bog-standard NHS old people's care home where they have no understanding of being gay, let alone HIV and AIDS.

I have a little dream that perhaps the gay community could get together and set up a sort of Chelsea Pensioners Home for those of us who fought in the war on HIV, who haven't had a chance to put money aside for our old age, where we could be looked after with dignity. Instead of red, like the Chelsea Pensioners, we'd all wear pink sparkly coats. But I don't think we really register in the millennial gay consciousness. All I hear of chem-sex and barebacking suggests the lessons we learned the hard way about safe sexuality have been put aside. I fear we've all been forgotten, this small handful of us who survived.

How did I survive? Perhaps I have some genetic quirk in my DNA. Or perhaps it was pure bloody-mindedness, a determination to keep the virus within me sleeping. I call it my sleeping dragon; you have to avoid anything that might ignite its fire and wake it up, like stress, like not looking after yourself, like eating badly. For me, in those days before combination therapy, survival was my daily work, making sure I didn't fall into the abyss psychologically or physically. I went back to creativity, would take a day trip to the beach and pick up found objects to turn into collages, which I called my Survival Art.

After Sam died, I got a little dog, a Belgian griffon called Totti, whom I named after a rather handsome Italian football player. I went on to breed these little griffons. I practised meditation and physical activities that would keep myself in harmony and keep the dragon asleep.

But most of all, it was a fierce desire to be sitting here so many years later, as I am, saying to the ghosts of those I once knew: I remember you, I'm going to tell your stories and keep your memory alive.

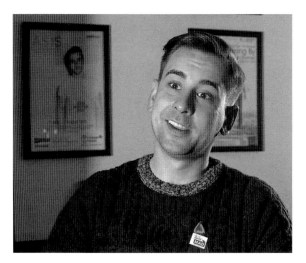

> "I know now I can still love and be loved, and that is the most precious gift in life."

Andrew Keates grew up on a council estate in Dorset and came out as gay at the age of 13. Always drawn to the theatre, he is now a multi-award-winning theatre director, many of whose productions have found their way to the West End, including William Hoffman's AIDS play *As Is*, the European première of *Dessa Rose* starring Cynthia Erivo and, in 2019, Michael Dennis's play, *Dark Sublime*. In 2018 the Vice Chancellor of Surrey University awarded him a Young Achiever of the Year Award, in recognition not only of his success in the theatre, but also of his work raising awareness of HIV and those from under-represented backgrounds.

> "At that moment I felt a little less alone. I understood I had a virus that affects all generations, all genders, all colours, all creeds."

Andrew's generation was failed by Section 28; the non-promotion of homosexuality in schools didn't provide them with any relevant sexual health education at a time, nor were there authentic gay role models in the media. Thanks to an overwhelming sense of shame, Andrew freely admits that as he came into adulthood there were times when he didn't care if he lived, let alone whether someone was wearing a condom. In 2013, after seeing HIV infection rates in London soar, he decided to direct a revival of William Hoffman's AIDS play As Is, *honouring all those who were lost to the AIDS pandemic whilst raising awareness about HIV today – giving others what he had lacked as a younger man. He had a pact with his cast and creative team that they would all have an HIV test. At the end of the production, he discovered he himself was positive.*

Andrew Keates
"All generations, all genders …"

I t never occurred to me for a moment that I was anything but negative. I sat in a room at the sexual health clinic, flirting and joking with a very attractive nurse, who took a small prick of blood from my finger and popped it into a little pot. Then he went quiet.

I saw his expression and said, "It's not positive, is it?"

He put his hand on my shoulder and said, "It is, mate, and we're going to look after you." I don't remember much about what happened next. I was in intense shock. In that moment my only thought as I reeled out onto the street was who do I tell? Whom can I ask for help? How can I phone my mum and tell her this, the one thing she was frightened of when I told her I was gay?

I was referred to a clinic at St Thomas's Hospital. I sat looking round the waiting room which was full of people: a mother with a baby, screaming its head off, a smart man in a grey suit, some old queens in their leather and plenty of young people. I longed to have some simple STD like chlamydia or gonorrhoea, which I presumed was what most of them had, waiting to be diagnosed.

When I went in to see the nurse, he quickly disabused me. "We don't do sexual screening in this clinic," he said. "Every single person in that waiting room is HIV positive." At that moment I felt a little less alone. I understood I had a virus that affects all generations, all genders, all colours, all creeds. That in any carriage on a tube train in London, as that nurse explained, you are guaranteed not to be the only person with HIV. But what people need to realise is that it's not those who know they are HIV+ that are passing the virus on. Anyone on effective medication has undetectable amounts of virus which cannot be passed on. It's the people who don't know, who may well be laughing the loudest and pointing the finger at others, who could be passing it on themselves.

Young people often downgrade the risk of AIDS and HIV because they imagine you take a pill and everything's fine. But that's not always the case.

"It sounds strange, but in many ways being HIV+ is the best thing that ever happened to me because it gave me a purpose and a reason to live."

In the first six months on medication – in my case it was Atripla – I lost two stone in weight. The days were like walking through cotton wool and the nights brought chronic insomnia, hallucinations and the worst night terrors you can imagine. My brain felt on fire. Every other day I had to change my sheets because either they were saturated in sweat or my bowels had relaxed. I accepted this state of affairs because I didn't realise there were other drugs out there, but fortunately my doctor took one look at me months later and realised I needed to change regime. That one wasn't ideal either, but eventually we arrived at the point of me being able to take a single pill every day that keeps my viral count undetectable and gives me a strong CD4 (T-cell count) reading so I know my immune system is relatively strong. Of course, no one can say how fine I will be in later years. The medication controls the virus, but it is not a cure.

I was tempted to keep the fact I was positive secret, because I feared the way others would treat me. But my mum had always brought me up to own who I am and be proud of it. I was already working with a charity in the theatre called the Make A Difference Trust, which builds awareness of HIV and AIDS and raises money for projects all over the world. They were holding an event at the Dominion Theatre in the West End, and I volunteered to go on stage and come out as being HIV+ to inspire others to get tested. Since that day I've been messaged by hundreds, thousands of people who have been afraid to reveal their status, thanking me for being open. It sounds strange, but in many ways being HIV+ is the best thing that ever happened to me because it gave me a purpose and a reason to live. The biggest obstacle for people with HIV isn't the virus. It's what everyone around them is saying and thinking.

And we have to change that because it denies them the most incredible experience, which is to fall in love and be with someone. Couples who once would have been separated through death are now separated through prejudice. The message we have to get across is that with today's HIV medication and viral load testing – not to mention PrEP

– undetectable HIV equals untransmissible HIV, and serodiscordant couples can keep themselves safe and still enjoy sex. I know now I can still love and be loved, and that is the most precious gift in life.

"The biggest obstacle for people with HIV isn't the virus. It's what everyone around them is saying and thinking. And we have to change that…"

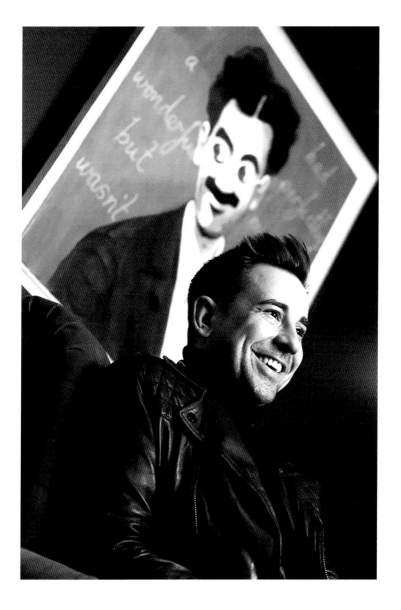

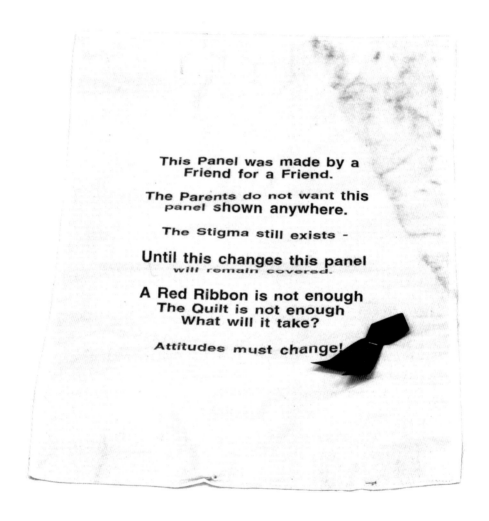

Detail from one of the quilt panels collected by the AIDS Memorial Quilt Preservation Partnership.

Afterword
Nick Thorogood

The future of HIV should be very different to its past.

Now in countries where drugs are both available and affordable, most people who are HIV-positive can manage their condition with a regime as simple as one pill a day, with life expectancy in line with the general population. An HIV positive person who is being treated with effective medication and whose viral load has become undetectable is unable to pass on the virus during sex. This is often referred to as U=U (undetectable equals untransmissible).

People at high risk can protect themselves with PrEP (pre-exposure prophy-laxis) which is a pill that can be taken by HIV-negative people before sex that reduces the risk of getting HIV. For people who may have put themselves at risk (e.g. through unprotected sex), PEP (post-exposure prophylaxis) taken within 72 hours can stop an HIV infection after the virus has entered a person's body. Meanwhile a United Nations initiative aims to bring an end to the AIDS pandemic by 2030 – a fast track programme with a big ambition.

The threat and fear of HIV in the present day is very different to the 1980s.

However, we must not forget the past – there are still millions of people whose lives have been affected in some way by HIV/AIDS, and you have read some of those stories in this book. We are very grateful that people have been brave enough to share their very personal testimony both here in print and also in our filmed interviews. At the National HIV Story Trust we believe much can be learnt from our recent past, and that we can build on these experiences as we face new pandemics and medical crises.

It is sad that already the HIV/AIDS pandemic, the fear, the outrage, the prejudice and the amazing acts of kindness and care are being forgotten – ask a teenager what they know about HIV and their knowledge will be sketchy at best – and if we forget this recent past, how can we learn from it?

Our charity is focused on education – keeping history alive by sharing the many personal stories we have gathered through people's own voices – in a filmed archive of over 150 hours. Through creating films, working with theatres, holding seminars for students and the public, and now publishing this, our first book, we are determined that whatever can be learnt from the last 40 years is told, retold and can benefit future generations. www.nhst.org.uk

The NHST is a registered charity, funded by donations and staffed entirely by volunteers. We welcome any support in the work we do – donations, skills and ideas. If you would like to help us please contact us at contact@nhst.org.uk.

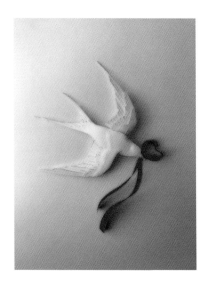

Index

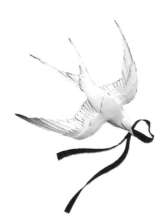